Treatment
of Carpal Tunnel Syndrome

Single Surgical Procedures **9**

A Colour Atlas of

Treatment of Carpal Tunnel Syndrome

W. Bruce Conolly

W DE G

Walter de Gruyter · Berlin · New York 1984

W. Bruce Conolly, FRCS, FRACS, FACS; Surgeon-in-charge, Sydney;
Hospital Hand Clinic, Sydney, Australia

Original Publishers: Wolfe Medical Publications Ltd., · London
Exclusive co-publishers for the Federal Republic of Germany and Austria:
Walter de Gruyter & Co., Genthiner Strasse 13, D-1000 Berlin 30. 1984.

Printed by Royal Smeets Offset b.v., Weert, Netherlands

Cover design: Rudolf Hübler

General Editor, Wolfe Surgical Atlases:
William F. Walker, DSc, ChM, FRCS (Eng.), FRCS (Edin.), FRS (Edin.)

CIP-Kurztitelaufnahme der Deutschen Bibliothek

Conolly, W. Bruce:
A colour atlas of treatment of carpal tunnel syndrome/
W. Bruce Conolly. -
Berlin; New York: de Gruyter, 1984.
(Single surgical procedures; 9)
ISBN 3-11-010098-3
ISBN 3-11-010099-1 (Subskr.-Pr.)
NE: GT

Part A Carpal tunnel syndrome: general principles

Contents

Part B Carpal tunnel decompression (and related procedures) – surgical techniques

Contents

Acknowledgements

I would like to express my appreciation to those many colleagues who have helped me in the preparation of this book. I am particularly indebted to Dr Ian Isaacs for his considerable help and advice. I also extend my gratitude to doctors C.C. McKellar, D.G. Gronow, P.G. Greenwell, M.K. Senapati, M. Perko, R. Garrick, and D. Bokor.

My thanks go to Mr Reg Money and Mr Peter Holloman for their photographic assistance, to Mr John Collins for the line drawings, and Ms Judith Maundrell and Susan Richards for library research assistance. I thank Miss Margaret Fitzgerald and Mrs Melissa Staples for their secretarial assistance.

Finally, my sincere gratitude goes to Miss Eveline Gallard for her infinite patience in preparing the manuscript, and her willingness to perform countless other tasks necessary in the preparation of this book.

This book is dedicated to

The Sydney Hospital Hand Unit, its patients and each member of its staff and my family:
Joyce, John, Christine, and Bruce

Introduction

The 'carpal tunnel syndrome' is a common hand condition. It is seen in many fields of medicine – general practice, general, plastic and orthopaedic surgery, internal medicine, rheumatology, etc. It is also seen by hand therapists, splint-makers, *et al.*

Surgical treatment is indicated in about 40 per cent of patients with this syndrome. Although the procedure is regarded as a simple one, there are complications which can lead to a disability far greater than the original complaint.

This book is divided into two parts: Part A outlines the general features of carpal tunnel syndrome; Part B illustrates a commonly practised method of operative treatment.

Definition and synonyms

The 'carpal tunnel syndrome' is also known as *compression neuropathy of the median nerve in the carpal tunnel, tardy median palsy* (when the palsy follows some time after trauma), *median neuropathy,* and *thenar atrophy.*

The syndrome results from compression of the median nerve within the carpal tunnel. Any condition which reduces the capacity of the carpal tunnel may compress the median nerve and so cause the syndrome; the commonest cause is swelling or thickening of the flexor tenosynovium. The terms 'spontaneous median neuropathy' or 'idiopathic median neuropathy' are used when there is no discernible cause.

The syndrome occurs in adults of any age, but most often in those 30 to 60 years of age. Its occurrence in childhood is rare(64). It is five times more common in females than males(83), and occurs more frequently in the dominant hand though both hands are often involved.

Historical aspects

1854 Paget(80) described compression of the median nerve at the wrist secondary to trauma.
1895 Jones described 'numbness and weakness' in middle aged women(47).
1910 Hunt(41) described occupational neuritis of the thenar branch of the median nerve.
1913 Marie and Foix(69) demonstrated neuromata in both median nerves just proximal to the 'transverse ligament' at the autopsy of a patient with thenar muscle atrophy. There was no history of injury. They were probably the first to recommend decompression of the median nerve by section of the transverse carpal ligament.
1930 Learmonth(63) decompressed the 'anterior annular ligament' in a patient with carpal tunnel syndrome, secondary to osteoarthritis of the wrist.
1938 Moersch(76) recommended section of the 'transverse carpal ligament' in a patient with bilateral median neuritis. No operation was performed.
1946 Cannon and Love(14) reported on 38 cases of tardy median nerve palsy. Nine patients were treated by section of the transverse carpal ligament.
1947 Brain, Wright and Wilkinson(9) described spontaneous compression of the median nerve in the carpal tunnel. They reported six patients treated successfully by sectioning of the 'transverse carpal ligament'.
1947 Phalen(85) reported four cases of carpal tunnel syndrome, three of whom were treated surgically.
1966 Phalen(82) reported on 654 hands with carpal tunnel syndrome in 439 patients.

The 'anterior annular ligament' and the 'transverse carpal ligament' are the same anatomical structure as the flexor retinaculum.

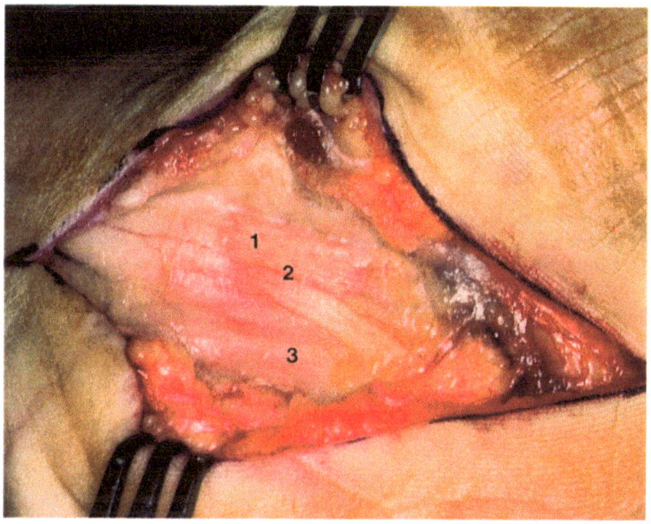

1 Operative findings in a patient with carpal tunnel syndrome. The median nerve (1) is congested and slightly compressed by the flexor retinaculum. There is continuity of the median artery (2). There appears to be a significant amount of tenosynovium (3).

Anatomy (see also pages 40–44)

The **carpal tunnel** is a rigid osteoligamentous canal bounded by the flexor retinaculum anteriorly and the carpal bones posteriorly (see **3**).

The **flexor retinaculum** (also known as the transverse carpal ligament, the annular or anterior annular ligament) is a thick (2 to 4 mm) rigid fibrous sheet stretching across the cavity of the carpal arch. It is attached on the ulnar side to the pisiform bone and the hook of the hamate, and radially to the tubercle of the scaphoid and the tubercle of the trapezium (see **2, 3, 23, 24, 25**).

At its attachment to the trapezium it divides into two parts, one of which is attached to the tubercle of the trapezium and the other to the medial part of the palmar surface of the bone, dorsal to the groove that lodges the tendon of the flexor carpi radialis. This attachment converts the groove of the flexor radialis tendon into a special tunnel through which the tendon proceeds to the floor of the carpal canal, to reach its insertion at the base of the 2nd metacarpal (see **3**).

At its upper border the flexor retinaculum is continuous with the deeper layer of deep fascia at the wrist – that which lies behind the flexor carpi ulnaris, flexor carpi radialis and palmaris longus muscles, but anterior to the other muscles (see **60, 61**).

Superficially it has fused to it the distal edge of the **volar carpal ligament**, except where the ulnar nerve and vessels separate these two layers, and on the superficial surface of its distal part it has attached to it fibres of the palmar aponeurosis and of the palmaris longus tendon, as these contribute to the palmar aponeurosis (see **3**).

Medially and laterally it gives origin to many of the muscles of the hypothenar and thenar eminences.

The **volar carpal ligament** is a variable thickening of transverse fibres in the superficial layer of the deep fascia of the forearm at the wrist (the layer of fascia lying anterior to the palmaris longus and the flexor carpi radialis and ulnaris muscles). It is attached radially to the styloid process of the radius and on the ulnar side to the styloid process of the ulna and the pisiform bone. Its lower border is indistinct, fusing with the anterior surface of the upper part of the flexor retinaculum, except over the ulnar nerve and vessels.

2 Diagram of nerves and vessels of the hand in relation to bones and skin markings.

2

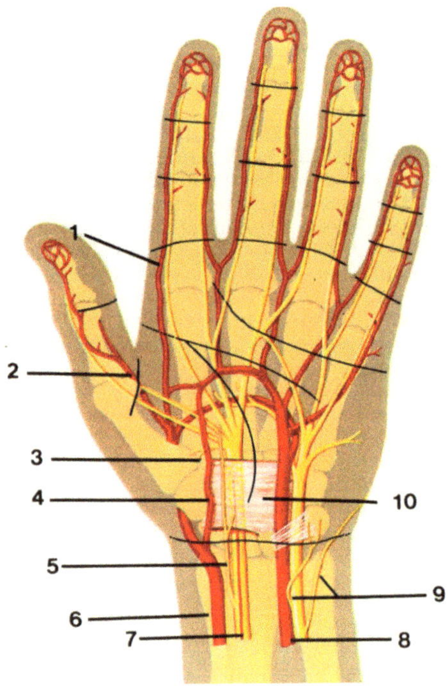

3

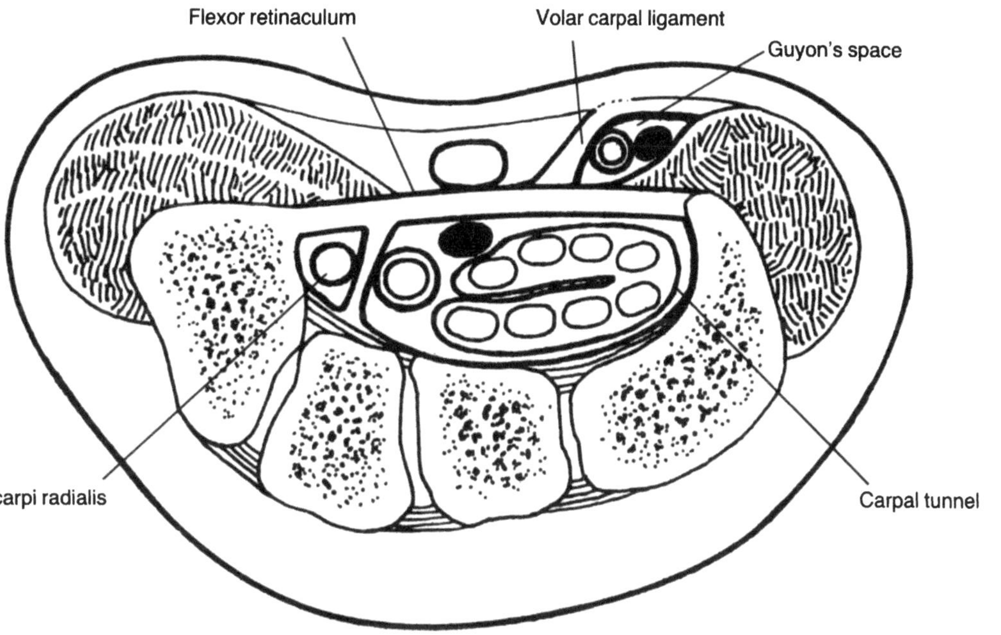

3 Diagrammatic transverse section through the mid-carpus showing the flexor retinaculum and the three 'canals' (see also **77**) i.e. carpal tunnel, Guyon's space, flexor carpi radialis tunnel.

Figure 2

1 Radialis indicis artery
2 Princeps pollicis artery
3 Branch to muscles of thumb
4 Superficial palmar artery
5 Median nerve and its palmar branch
6 Radial artery
7 Median artery
8 Ulnar artery
9 Ulnar nerve and dorsal branch
10 Flexor retinaculum

ANATOMY

The carpal tunnel is incapable of accommodating much increase in its tissue content without the median nerve being forced up against the firm inelastic flexor retinaculum, causing motor and sensory changes in the median nerve distally. The commonest cause is swelling or thickening of the tenosynovium surrounding the nine flexor tendons(67).

At the distal end of the carpal tunnel the median nerve divides into a lateral division, giving rise to the recurrent motor branch and three proper palmar digital nerves to the thumb and index finger, and a medial division, giving rise to two common palmar digital nerves to the 2nd and 3rd clefts, and a constant communicating branch to the ulnar digital branches(98).

There are considerable variations in the palmar cutaneous, motor, and digital sensory branches. There are also variations in the course of the median nerve itself. It occasionally has a high division and occasionally a low division into its divisions or branches; there may be a persisting median artery.

Thus there are **three canals**, the **carpal canal proper**, **the canal for flexor carpi radialis**, and **Guyon's space** (see **3**). The floor of this space is the flexor retinaculum and some fibres of the muscles of the hypothenar eminence. The multi-layered oblique roof consists of the volar carpal ligament that blends distally with the hypothenar fascia, radially with the palmar aponeurosis, and proximally with the deep fascia of the forearm. The palmaris brevis also contributes to the roof. The vertical ulnar wall comprises the flexor carpi ulnaris, the pisiform bone and the abductor digiti minimi.

Guyon(37) gave, as the dimensions of his space or loge, 1 cm or 1.5 cm in all directions. The loge contains the ulnar artery and nerve.

Ten structures pass through the carpal tunnel: the median nerve, the flexor pollicis longus tendon, and the eight flexor tendons to the four fingers. The tendons are enveloped by the synovium of the radial and ulnar bursa. There is a large potential space between the visceral and parietal layers of these bursae.

The median nerve is the softest and most volar structure in the carpal tunnel. It lies directly beneath the flexor retinaculum and superficial to the nine digital flexor tendons. The median nerve courses through the tunnel within a thin perineural sheath which merges imperceptibly with the flexor tenosynovium.

4a

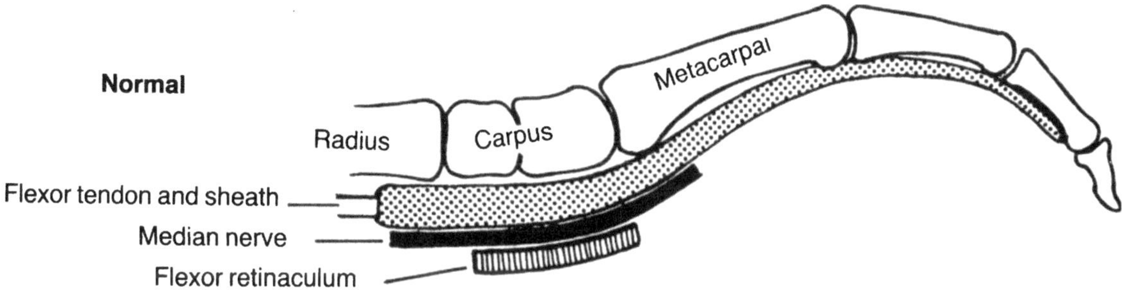

4b

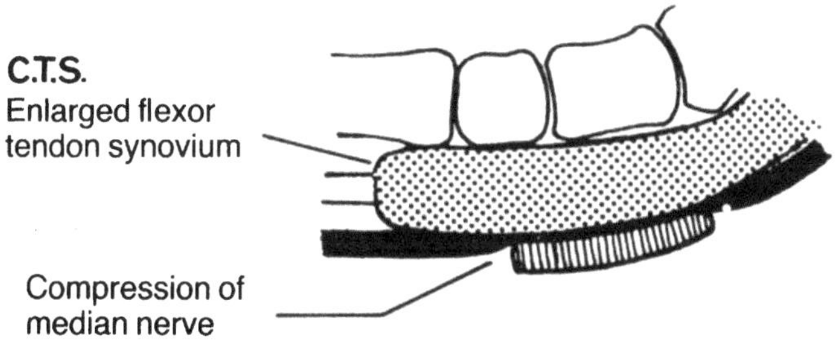

4a and b Sagittal view of the carpal tunnel.
(4a) The normal.
(4b) Compression of the median nerve beneath the flexor retinaculum by enlarged flexor tenosynovium i.e. CTS.

Pathogenesis [97, 98, 99]

1 Course of the median nerve. Near the wrist the median nerve comes from the deep surface of the superficialis (formerly called sublimis) to which it adheres, and winds around the radial side of the tendon of the index finger onto the palmar aspect. If this tendon has muscular fibres extending to the distal forearm, the median nerve can be irritated by the action of this muscle tendon unit.

2 The median nerve is the softest and most volar structure in the carpal tunnel. It lies directly beneath the flexor retinaculum and superficial to the nine digital flexor tendons. The carpal tunnel is incapable of accommodating much increase in its tissue content without the median nerve being forced up against the firm inelastic flexor retinaculum, causing motor and sensory changes in the median nerve distally.

The commonest cause of carpal tunnel syndrome is swelling or thickening of the tenosynovium surrounding the nine flexor tendons.

3 Longitudinal glide of the median nerve. With full finger flexion the median nerve glides proximally under the flexor retinaculum; with full finger extension the median nerve glides distally[73]. Tethering of the nerve in the carpal tunnel may be responsible for pain radiating proximally up the median nerve.

4 Tension and pressures in the carpal tunnel. Tension of the flexor tendons produced by forcible digital and wrist flexion causes impingement of the median nerve against the flexor retinaculum[1]. Flexion of the wrist causes increased pressure in the proximal part of the carpal tunnel. Extension of the wrist causes increased pressure in the distal part of the carpal tunnel[102].

Thus repetitive hand activities involving pinch or grasp during wrist flexion may be a contributing factor in some instances of carpal tunnel syndrome[95].

Note: The capacity of the carpal tunnel is least at its mid-point and is further reduced by extreme positions of flexion or extension of the wrist.

Table 1. Pressures in the carpal tunnel[30].

Wrist position	Control (12 patients)	Carpal tunnel syndrome (15 patients)
Neutral	2.5 mm Hg	32 mm Hg
Wrist flexion	31 mm Hg	94 mm Hg
Wrist extension	30 mm Hg	110 mm Hg

5 Microscopic factors(98). The number of funiculi in the median nerve in the carpal tunnel varies from 6 to 40 bundles, the average being 24. The funiculi occupy from one-third to two-thirds of the cross-sectional area. Although there is considerable variation, the connective tissue content of the median nerve in the tunnel may be two-thirds, thus providing a cushioning effect in the carpal tunnel.

Patients with larger and fewer funiculi and less connective tissue are probably more prone to carpal tunnel syndrome.

The perineurium is relatively thicker in the carpal tunnel than at other levels. It is elastic and resists and maintains intrafunicular pressure. The perineurium is not crossed by lymphatic vessels and therefore acts as a diffusion barrier.

There are only capillaries in the funiculus; the arteries and veins reside in the epineurium. The nutrient vessels take an oblique course through the perineurium. Thus there is a valvular mechanism, and any swelling of the funiculus blocks off the valve, leading to ischaemia of the funiculus.

6 Fluid retention. This plays a significant role in the precipitation of symptoms by increasing the volume of the flexor tenosynovium, and causes congestion of the median nerve. Fluid retention is maximal at night, waking the patient. Elevation and exercise, by reducing the fluid in the carpal tunnel, usually gives some relief.

7 Associated connective tissue disorders(67, 78, 83). These include flexor tenovaginitis, de Quervain's disease, epicondylitis, periarthritis of the shoulder, Raynaud's disease(66), and peripheral neuritis.

8 Multiple nerve lesions(105). Carpal tunnel syndrome can be associated with ulnar nerve entrapment. Pathological changes at one level may influence vulnerability at the other(68).

In patients with multiple entrapment neuropathies there may be no underlying systemic disorder, but associated metabolic disorders such as diabetes mellitus, rheumatoid disease, should be excluded.

Involvement of the ulnar nerve

The ulnar nerve in Guyon's space is better protected and not as easily injured as is the median nerve in the carpal tunnel(3). However, double tunnel nerve compression syndromes (carpal and Guyon's tunnel or space or loge syndrome have been reported in burns at the wrist(26)).

Table 2. Pathological changes* associated with nerve compression(16), (82)

Type of compression	Pathology	Effect on function
Transient, mild	Venous stasis leading to anoxia	The nerve recovers when the compression is relieved and the circulation restored
Sustained and increased	Local dispersal of myelin Conduction delay or block	Motor fibres more susceptible than sensory fibres
Prolonged, unrelieved	Wallerian degeneration Narrowing of nerve with intraneural fibrosis	Slow recovery after release of pressure Irreversible loss of function

*Two factors operate(81) 1 Direct pressure
2 Interference with blood supply

ACUTE CARPAL TUNNEL SYNDROME(4, 12, 71)

The acute carpal tunnel syndrome, though rare(3, 85) may be caused by:
1 Excessive hand exercise(102);
2 Oedema from injury(3) or operation, acute suppurative infection in the carpal tunnel, burns(26), acute rheumatoid arthritis, gout;
3 Dislocation of the lunate;
4 Haemorrhage into the carpal tunnel(42);
5 Thrombosis of an anomalous median artery(12);
6 Iatrogenic injection injury of the median nerve (see **20** to **22**).

5
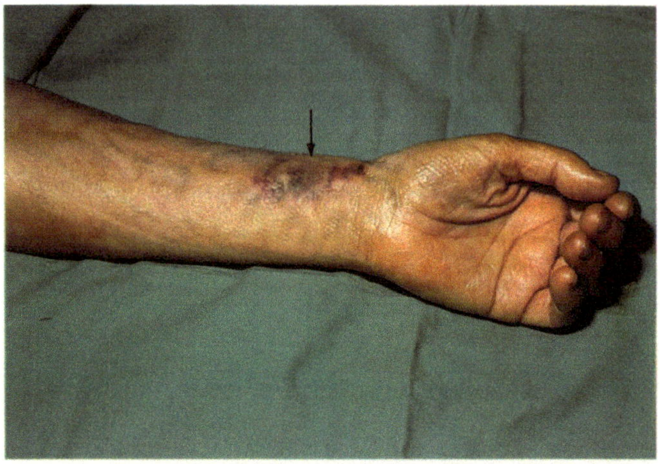

5 Acute carpal tunnel syndrome developed three days after cannulation of the radial artery. This 75-year-old man was being treated for cardiovascular collapse. Note the bruising around the site of cannulation (arrowed).

6
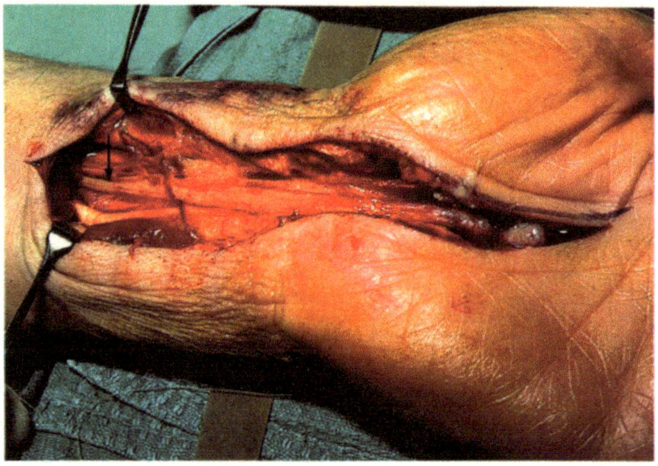

6 Operative finding. Thrombosis of the median artery. The arrow points to a 2 cm length of ischaemic nerve.

7

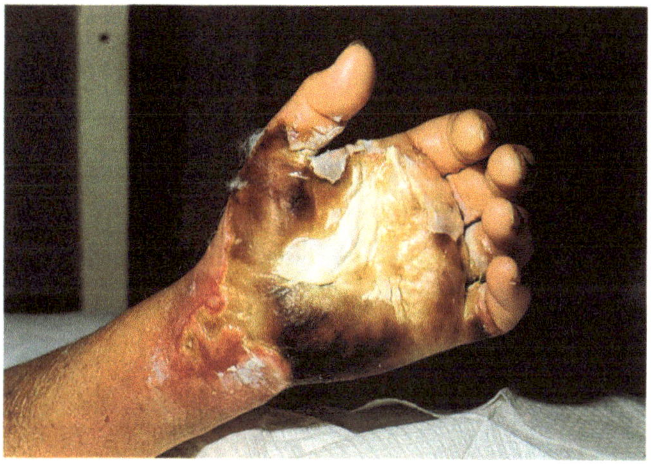

7 Acute carpal tunnel syndrome. A severe anaerobic infection developed after a minor laceration to the palm of a 55-year-old housewife. Oedema caused a severe acute carpal tunnel syndrome manifesting as pain and numbness in the median nerve distribution of her hand.

8

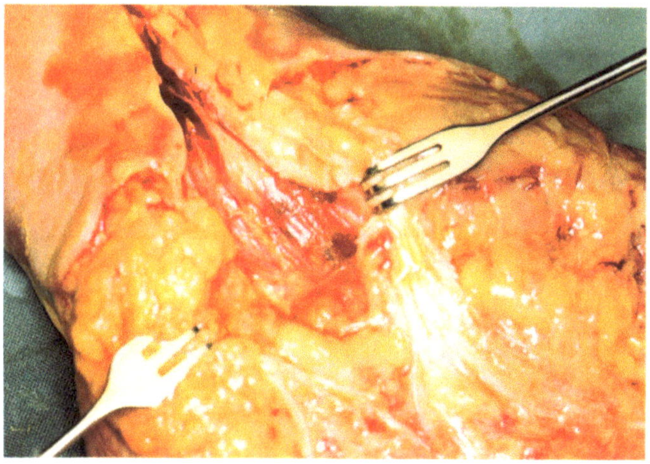

8 Operative findings. Severe compression of the median nerve with congestion and ischaemic necrosis.

Causes of carpal tunnel syndrome

9 The normal carpal tunnel. Diagram of walls and contents.

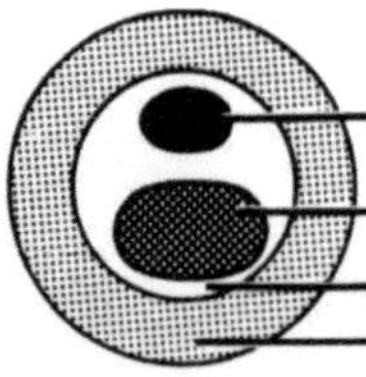

10 Carpal tunnel syndrome caused by increase in contents.

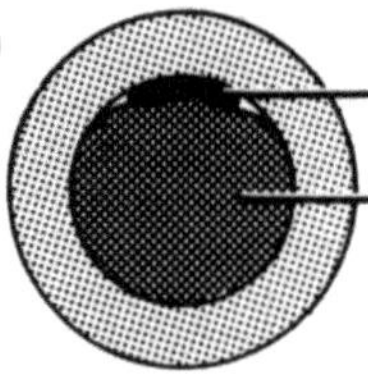

1 Increase in contents of the carpal tunnel[10]. This may be due to:

(a) Oedema or thickening of the flexor tenosynovium[43] e.g. flexor tenosynovitis, (rheumatoid[20, 83], traumatic[42], tuberculous[2, 43, 51]), chondromatosis[43].

(b) Odema from injury[42], infection[4], metabolic disorder[83].

(c) Space-occupying lesion
tumour (ganglion)[11], lipoma[8, 46], xanthoma, haemangioma[52], osteoid osteoma[39], anomalous intrinsic or extrinsic muscle bellies[102] (second lumbrical)[44], flexor superficialis indicis, palmaris profundus[6, 7].

(d) Deposits of gouty tophi[5, 107], calcium[70], etc.

(e) Haematoma – leukaemia[71], haemophilia[16].

11 Carpal tunnel syndrome caused by decrease in size of tunnel.

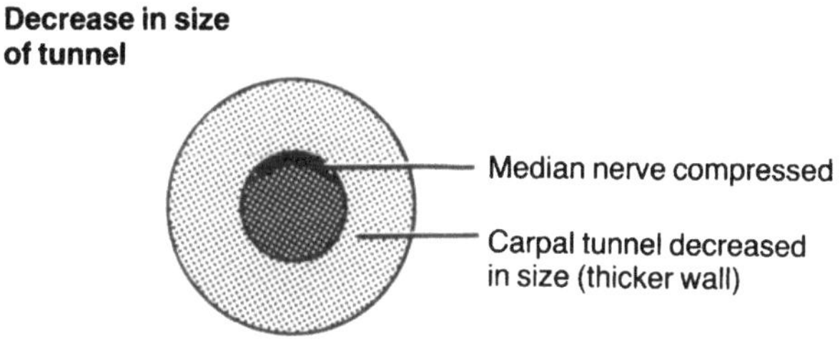

2 Decrease in size of the carpal tunnel[11]. This may be:

1 Transient or intermittent, for example, extremes of flexion or extension of the wrist[102].

2 Permanent (a) Bony floor – osteoarthritis[83], carpal dislocation (semi-lunar), Colles' fracture[42], etc. (b) Thickened flexor retinaculum from amyloid[57], acromegaly[90], myxoedema[42], etc. (c) Congenital narrowing of the carpal tunnel[23].

3 Miscellaneous conditions

These contribute to the carpal tunnel syndrome by increasing the content of the carpal tunnel (fluid, fat, amyloid, blood, etc.) or by decreasing the size of the carpal tunnel (carpal floor synovitis, acromegaly).

In diabetes and other neuropathies the median nerve is more susceptible to pressure; In leprosy the median nerve is enlarged; In disseminated lupus erythematosis the median nerve has an intrinsic vascular disorder.

(a) **Metabolic/endocrine** – rheumatoid disease, pregnancy, menopause, obesity, diabetes mellitus, thyrotoxicosis, myxoedema, gout, Raynaud's disease, multiple myeloma, amyloid, acromegaly.

(b) **Occupational aspects.** In occupations where there is repeated forceful flexion of the wrist and fingers there may be thick flexor tenosynovium and increased pressure in the carpal tunnel[102]; e.g. process work, laundry work, jack-hammer work, etc.

(c) **Median nerve conditions** – enlargement (leprosy, neurofibroma, lipoma), haemangioma or thrombosis of the median artery.

(d) **Familial**[24, 102].

Causes of carpal tunnel syndrome

Classification on an aetiological basis

Congenital
(a) Congenital narrowing of the carpal tunnel. Primary carpal stenosis.
(b) Anomalous intrinsic or extrinsic muscle bellies, for example, palmaris profundus.
(c) Extensive lumbrical or superficialis muscle bellies. Persistently large median artery.

Trauma
(a) Direct damage to bony carpal walls (carpal fracture or dislocation). In Colles' fracture immobilisation of the wrist in marked flexion and ulnar deviation may cause acute compression of the median nerve in the carpal tunnel immediately after reduction.
(b) Indirect damage causing oedema, insect sting[61], haematoma.
(c) Direct damage to the median nerve itself or indirect damage, leading to fibrosis and 'tardy median palsy'.
(d) Direct pressure from crutches or canes.

Infection
Acute suppurative infection.

Occupational
An occupation which increases the pressure in the carpal tunnel or by flexor tenosynovitis may predispose to the carpal tunnel syndrome.

Metabolic/endocrine
Endocrine imbalance, the most common of which is pregnancy[79, 110] especially the third trimester. Menopause, post-hysterectomy, post-öopherectomy. Contraceptive medication[89].

Inflammatory/degeneration
Rheumatoid disease, gout, amyloidosis, etc.

Tumour
Ganglion, lipoma, etc.

Vascular
Arterio-venous shunt (traumatic or surgical for renal dialysis[108]), Raynaud's disease, anomalous median artery[62, 83], spontaneous intraneural haemorrhage.

Changes in the median nerve

Even in cases of carpal tunnel syndrome where the symptoms are relieved by decompression, there is often no abnormality seen at operation[29, 82, 83]. Note that the normal median nerve flattens to some extent as it passes beneath the flexor retinaculum.

However, one or more of the following changes may occur, although the changes are not necessarily proportional to the severity of the symptoms[103].

Macroscopic

1 Hyperaemia and congestion, usually near the junction of the proximal and middle thirds of the flexor retinaculum.
2 Constriction.
3 Pseudoneuroma. This may be caused by oedema[83] or actual obstruction to axoplasm flow. The constriction should produce distal oedema.
4 Changes in the median artery, for example, enlargement, thrombosis.
5 Epineural adhesions.

Microscopic

1 Interfascicular fibrosis.
2 Loss of myelin sheath.
3 Axon constriction.

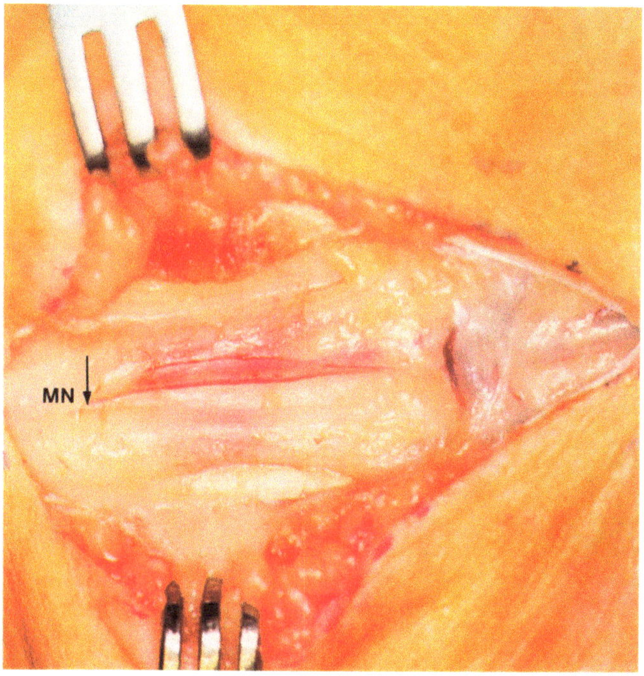

12

12 Congestion of the right median nerve (MN). Note the nerve has divided before it enters the carpal tunnel (arrow).

13

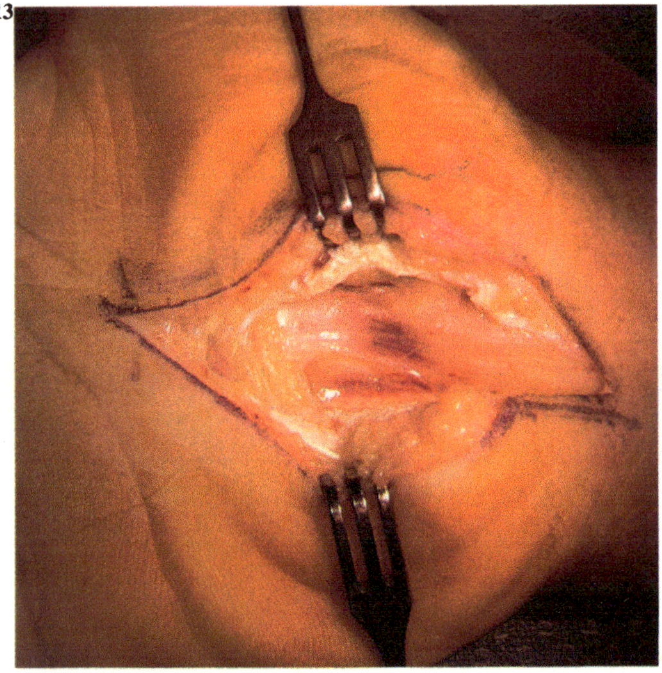

14

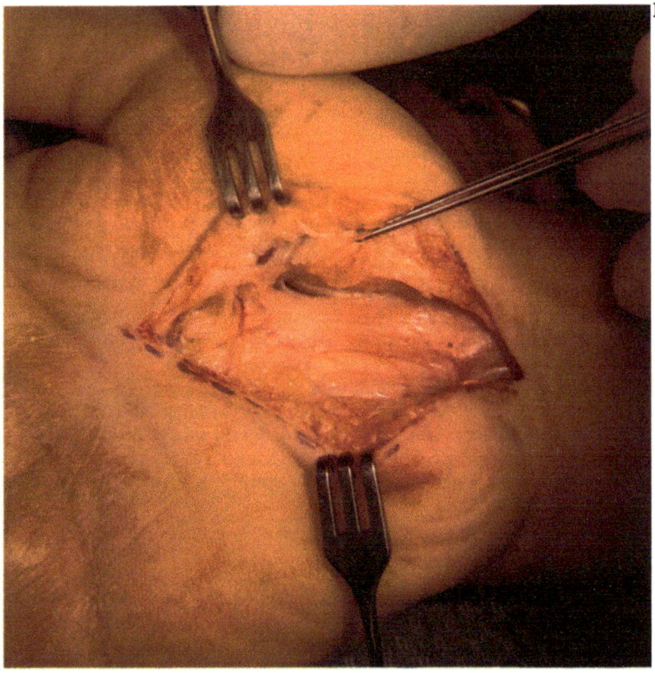

13 Severe congestion – right hand.

14 Congestion and constriction – right hand.

15

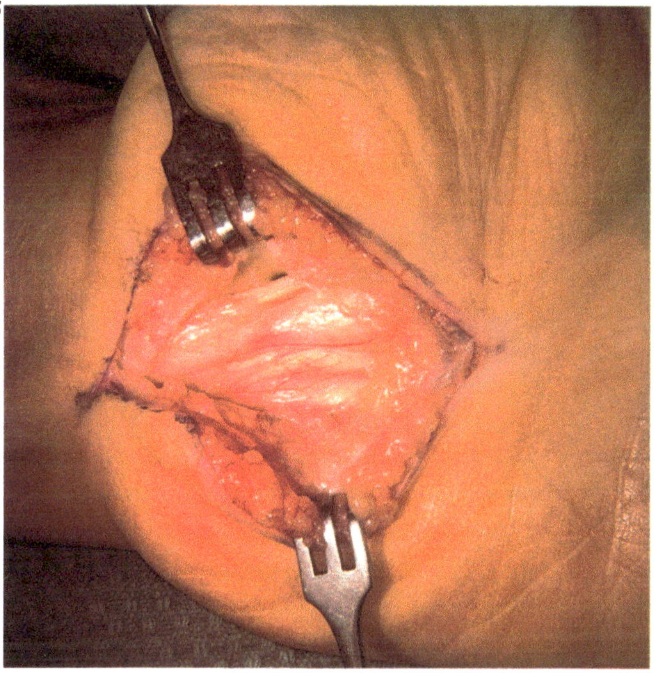

15 Constriction and pseudoneuroma formation – left hand.

16

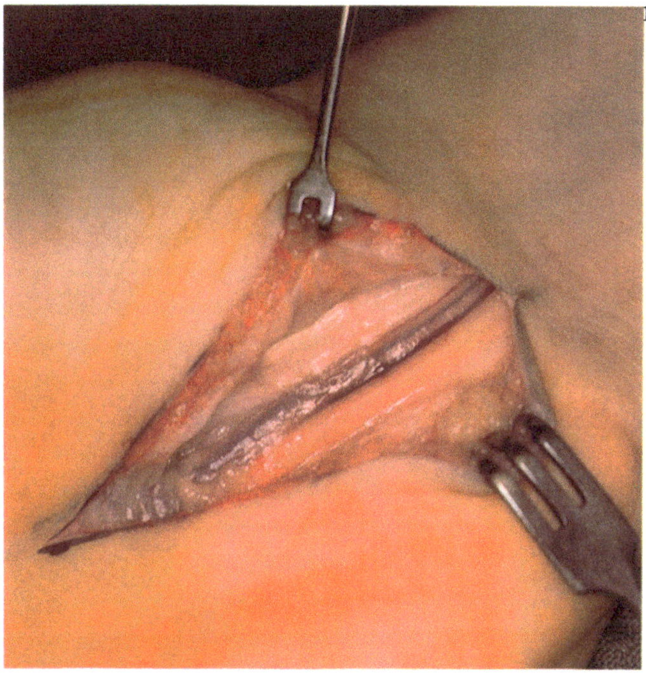

16 An abnormally large median artery lying between the two divisions of the median nerve – right hand. The median artery can be a major contributor to the blood supply of the hand and can cause carpal tunnel syndrome(62).

17

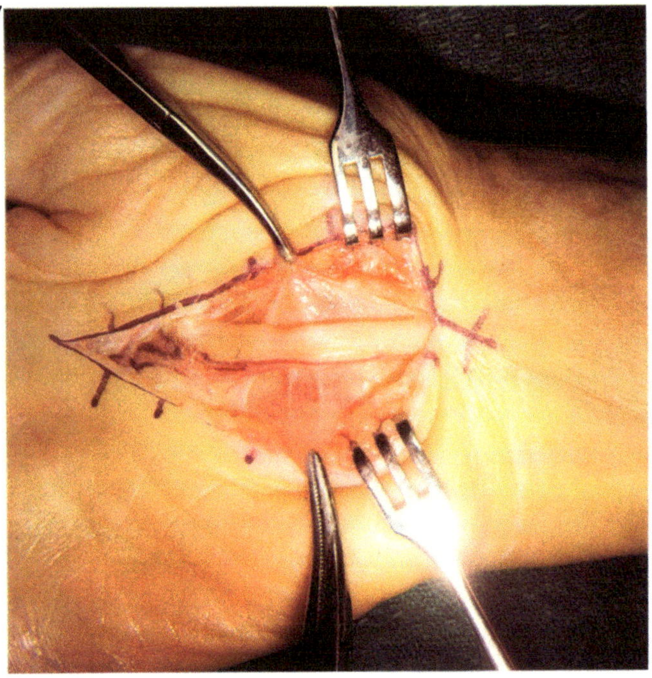

18

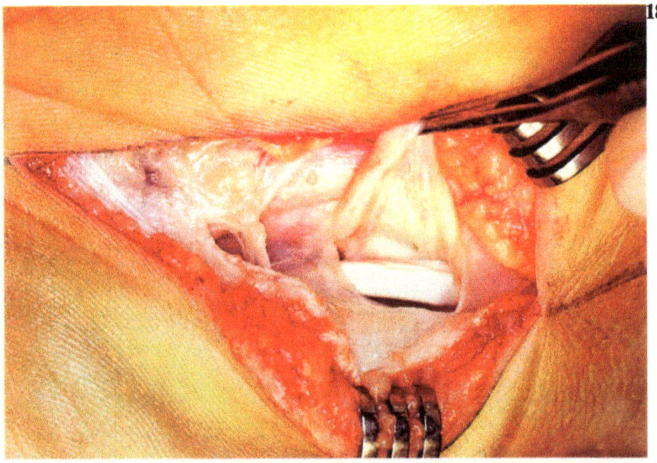

18 Proliferative flexor tenosynovitis obscuring and pressing on the median nerve. This patient worked as a labourer.

17 Thick epineurium, held by clamps.

19

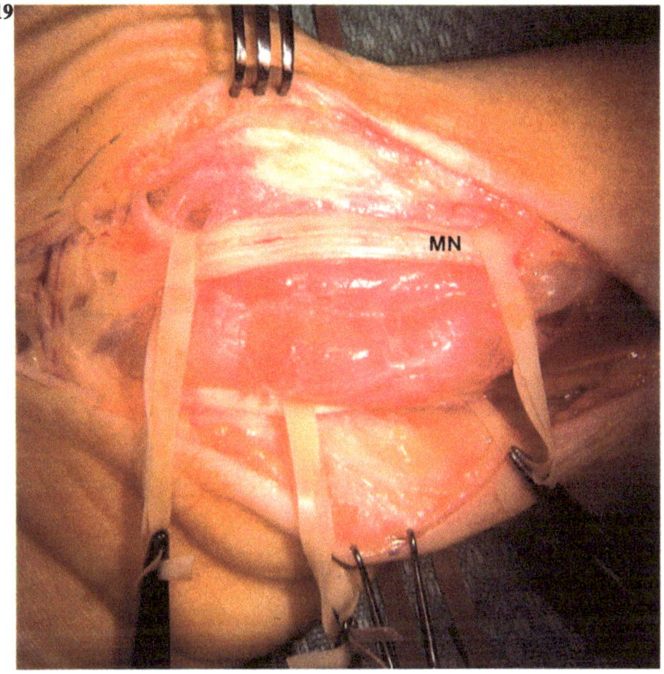

20

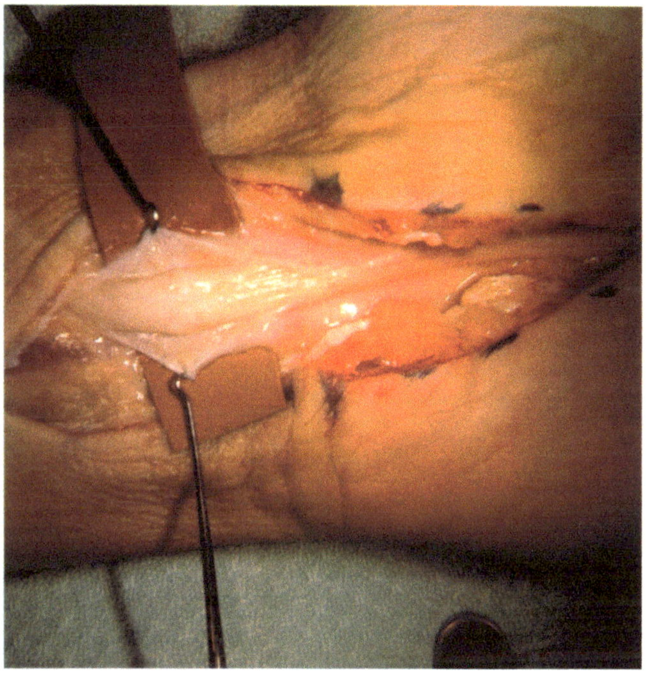

19 Rheumatoid involvement of the flexor tenosynovium causing compression of the median nerve (MN) in the carpal tunnel.

20 Epineural and intraneural fibrosis. This followed intraneural injection of local anaesthetic.

21

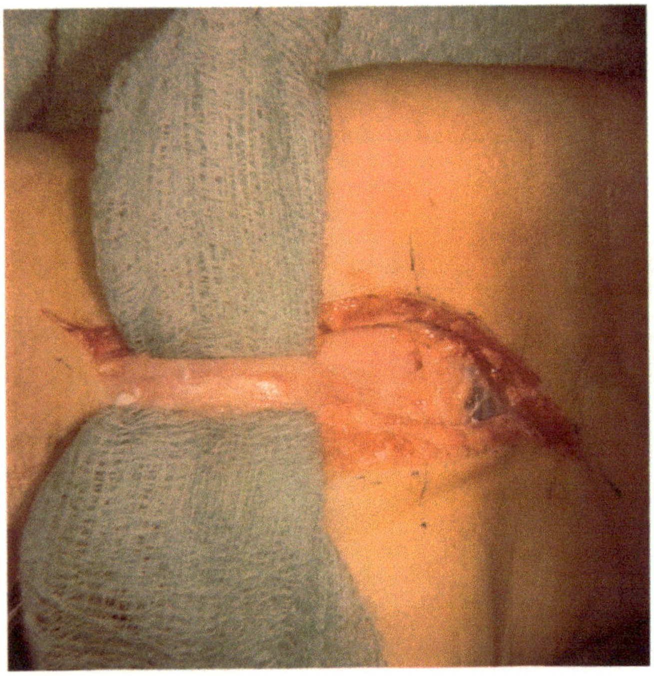

22

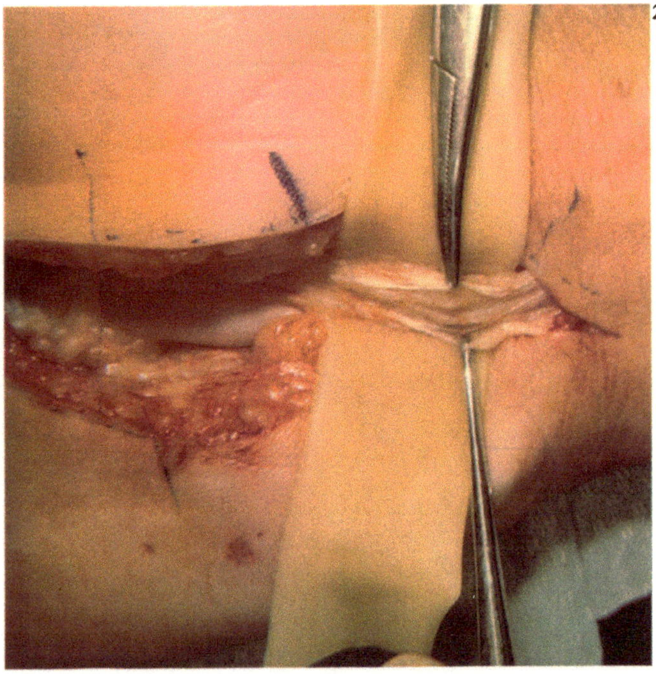

21 Cortisone infiltration and deposits from intraneural injection of cortisone.

22 Intraneural fibrosis after cortisone was injected into the median nerve.

Clinical features

Types

A carpal tunnel syndrome may present as an **acute**, a **chronic**, an **acute on chronic**, or as an **intermittent condition**.

The syndrome may be **mild, moderate** or **severe** and be **partial** or **total** in median nerve distribution.

The clinical features may be predominantly **sensory** or **motor** (with progressive thenar wasting without pain or numbness). Mostly there is a combination of sensory and motor symptoms and signs. Associated **autonomic** changes may be present.

Symptoms

Numbness, pain, and paraesthesia occur in the distribution of the median nerve in the hand, often associated with clumsiness, weakness of pinch, and difficulty in fine movements such as sewing and knitting. Sensory changes, both subjective and objective, may precede weakness and wasting often by weeks or months.

Characteristically, pain and paraesthesia are most distressing at night. The reasons for these nocturnal symptoms include: vasodilatation with vasoconstriction and oedema from carbon-dioxide retention during sleep, delayed venous return from impairment of the muscle pump in the arm, and pressure on the median nerve from wrist flexion or lying on the arm.

Most patients wake from sleep in the early hours of the morning with painful burning, numbness or tingling sensations in the fingers and hand. The discomfort is often not restricted to the hand, but may radiate up the arm to the shoulder and neck or chest. Pain proximal to the wrist may be caused by restricted longitudinal glide of the median nerve in the neck or upper limb. Alternatively, such pain may be caused by a co-existent cervical radiculopathy(17, 105). These symptoms are relieved by hanging the hand and arm over the side of the bed or getting up and walking about or shaking or exercising the hand. This is referred to as 'waking numbness'.

The fingers may feel swollen and the whole arm heavy. Clumsiness may be caused by sensory or motor impairment.

Because of the communications between the median and ulnar nerves, the symptoms may also involve the ring and little fingers, although predominantly the radial three digits are affected.

Simultaneous compression of the ulnar nerve in Guyon's space is rare. If there are sensory changes in the little finger one should look proximal to the wrist, usually the elbow or cervical spine(83).

Onset

Strenuous hand activity mostly aggravates the symptoms, although the numbness and tingling may not be noted until the hand has been resting for several hours after the activity.

Signs

There may be no objective findings in the early stages[83]. In these patients the diagnosis can usually be made on the history alone. Mostly there will be one or other physical signs, consistent with compression of the median nerve in the carpal tunnel. Abnormal signs proximal to the wrist would suggest a more proximal lesion.

Inspect and palpate the median nerve for a localised or a generalised swelling of the nerve, pulsations or tenderness.

Abnormal sensory findings include:

1 Impaired sensation to touch in the median nerve distribution of the fingers. Altered sensation in the distribution of the palmar branch in the proximal palm indicates a more proximal lesion, for example, compression beneath the pronator teres. Stroke lightly the palmar skin from fingertip to wrist. Patients with carpal tunnel syndrome often feel numbness in the fingertip, but have normal feeling in the palm.

2 Phalen's wrist test[83]. Unforced complete flexion of the wrist for 30 to 60 seconds produces paraesthesia in the median-nerve distribution in about 80 per cent of cases.

Have the patient place the backs of the hands against one another and flex the wrists fully.

The reverse Phalen test may be positive when the Phalen wrist flexion test is negative. Place the palms of the hands together and raise the elbows, thus extending the wrists and placing the median nerve on the stretch.

3 Tinel's sign. Tingling in one or more digits, elicited by gentle tapping of the median nerve at the wrist, is present in about 60 per cent of cases.

4 The tourniquet test[27, 34, 42, 106]. Inflation of a blood pressure cuff around the upper arm to above systolic pressure, or midway between systolic and diastolic pressure, often reproduces pain and paraesthesiae within 60 seconds. Sensory impairment can be detected within 10 minutes. The basis of this test lies in the increased susceptibility of the median nerve in the carpal tunnel to ischaemia or venous stasis.

Abnormal motor signs include:

1 Thenar muscle weakness, wasting or even paralysis; test this by forcible tip-to-tip pinch between the thumb and ring finger.
2 There may be weakness of lumbrical action to the middle finger.
3 Sometimes there is tenderness over the thenar motor branch.

Abnormal autonomic findings

The median nerve transmits most of the sympathetic nerve supply to the hand[1]. Abnormal findings may include:
(a) Discoloration of the skin.
(b) Disorder of sweating in the hand and fingers.
(c) Changes in the nail, for example, fragility, brittleness, shedding, etc.

Abnormal findings at the wrist

There may be swelling, with or without crepitus of the flexor tendons proximal to the carpal tunnel.

Variability in motor and sensory findings of median nerve compression may be caused by variations in the median and ulnar nerve and communications between them.

Miscellaneous findings[83]

There may also be the findings of co-existing conditions such as osteoarthritis, rheumatoid arthritis, Raynaud's disease[66], Dupuytren's disease, de Quervain's condition, trigger finger, tennis elbow, or periarthritis of the shoulder, cervical spondylosis, etc.

Clinical features

Symptoms	Pain and paraesthesia* 'Waking numbness' Clumsiness and weakness* Swelling and heaviness Sensitivity to cold
Signs in the hand	**Sensory** Impaired sensation† Positive Tinel's sign† Positive Phalen wrist flexion test† Tourniquet test
	Motor Thenar muscle weakness and wasting Lumbrical weakness to the middle finger
	Autonomic – vasomotor disorder Colour changes Sweat and nail changes
Other signs	**Wrist** Swelling of flexor tenosynovium proximal to the wrist Deformity from fracture or arthritis
	General Rheumatoid arthritis and osteoarthritis Acromegaly and other associated conditions

*In the early stages these symptoms occur in the morning and pass off during the day, unless the patient engages in heavy or repetitive manual activity, particularly with the wrist flexed. In the later stages they persist throughout the day.
†These tests are positive in two-thirds of patients, but none of these tests is absolutely diagnostic.

> The diagnosis of carpal tunnel syndrome should be considered in any patient with paraesthesiae in the median nerve distribution of the hand, or weakness or wasting of abductor pollicis brevis or opponens pollicis.

> The symptoms and signs of carpal tunnel syndrome may be obscured by the presence of other associated or unrelated conditions, e.g. rheumatoid arthritis, diabetes mellitus, etc[25].

Investigations

1 Xray
Arrange xray in any patient where there is the possibility of a skeletal derangement, which might precipitate or be associated with the carpal tunnel syndrome.
• Xray view of the carpal tunnel may show a bony tumour in the floor of the carpal tunnel.
• Xray of the hand and wrist may show associated arthritis or a previous fracture.
• Xray of the cervical spine may show cervical spondylosis, cervical rib, etc.

23

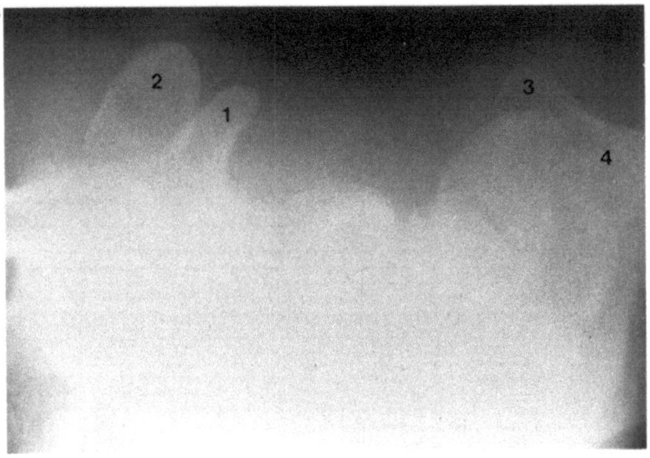

23 A normal carpal tunnel view. Note the four pillars of the carpal tunnel. 1 Hook of hamate; 2 Pisiform; 3 Tubercle of scaphoid; 4 Crest of trapezium. These are all palpable.

24

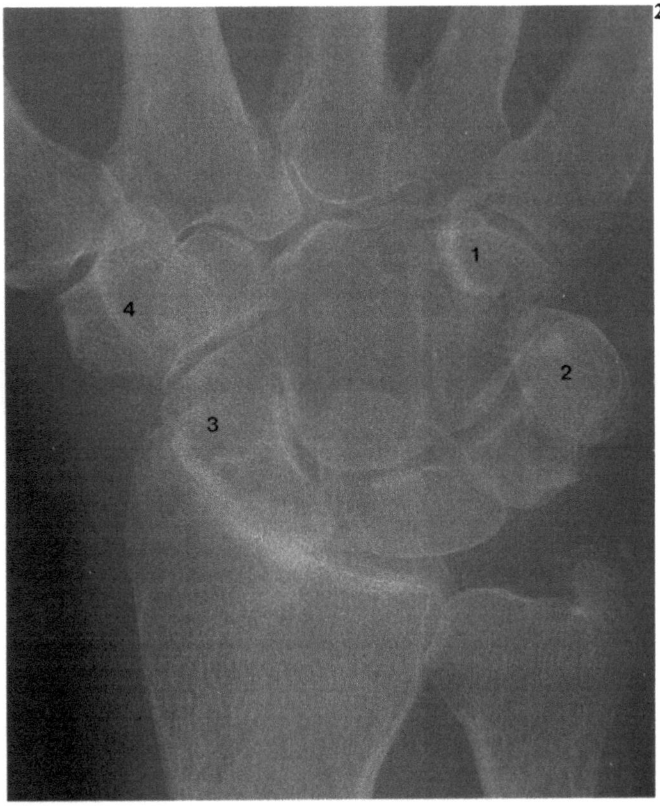

24 Posterior/anterior view. This patient had radiocarpal arthritis contributing to carpal tunnel syndrome.

24a

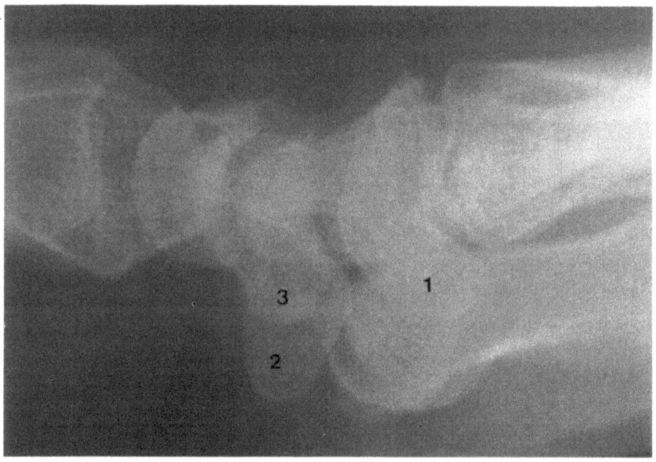

24a A normal lateral view. Note the pillars of the carpal tunnel.

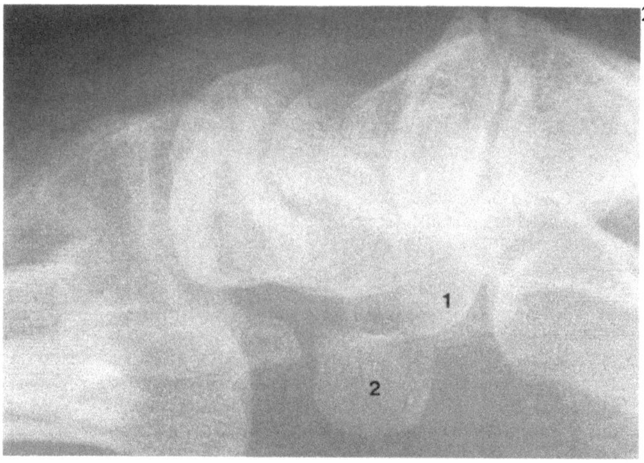

24b

24b Lateral view of a patient with acute carpal tunnel syndrome developing after a Colles' fracture, with displacement of the lower end of the radius.

2 Electromyography (EMG)
Most patients with carpal tunnel syndrome can be diagnosed on history alone. When both symptoms and signs provide clearcut evidence of carpal tunnel syndrome an EMG is unnecessary(80). There are times, however, when an EMG is useful in differentiating carpal tunnel syndrome from its simulators (see differential diagnosis, page 30). An EMG can save a patient from an unnecessary operation.

An EMG can help answer these questions(91).
1 Is there an organic lesion present?
2 Where is that lesion? Anterior horn cell, nerve or muscle?

EMG testing of muscles may reveal the presence of denervation before actual atrophy of muscles is observed clinically.
3 If it is in the nerve is it a generalised disorder or confined to one nerve?
4 If confined to one nerve (e.g. median nerve) can the lesion be localised e.g. to the carpal tunnel or more proximally?
In cervical spondylosis, normal latencies are often noted, but signs of denervation or proximal conduction (F wave) impairment will be present.
5 How severe is the median nerve involvement?
6 If there has been decompression is the nerve recovering, and if so, is the recovery progressive?
Following decompression there is improvement in motor and sensory conduction, although they may not return completely to normal values(35).

Motor latency. The normal motor latency is below about 4.4 milliseconds, depending on age. A latency of more than 5 milliseconds is suggestive of a carpal tunnel syndrome with moderate nerve damage. An increase to 6 or 7 milliseconds is considered to be an indication for immediate surgical intervention(36).

Delay in *sensory conduction* and reduced amplitude of sensory action potential also occurs and is a more sensitive indicator than motor latency(29). The upper limit of the normal range of latency to the peak of sensory action potential in the median nerve is about 4 milliseconds, and the lower limit of the normal range of amplitude is about 8 microvolts, depending on age.

In carpal tunnel syndrome an EMG is abnormal in about 50–80 per cent of cases(83, 91). A normal EMG does not rule out the diagnosis of a carpal tunnel syndrome.

The *diagnostic yield* from electromyography and nerve conduction studies may be significantly increased by various techniques such as comparing the affected side with the unaffected side, and by comparing the amplitude of median and ulnar sensory action potential. Specialised techniques may also be used in which delays in motor latency may be traced across the carpal tunnel.

Abnormalities of *ulnar nerve sensory action potential* are often found in carpal tunnel syndrome. In such patients a generalised sub-clinical neuropathy may be present(91).

3 Other tests
Other tests for diabetes, rheumatoid arthritis, gout, thyroid or other systemic problems are arranged as necessary.

Differential diagnosis

The following neurological conditions may mimic a carpal tunnel syndrome.

1 **Cervical cord and nerve root:** cervical spondylosis†, herniated disc, spinal cord tumour, progressive muscular atrophy, syringomyelia, disseminated sclerosis, thoracic outlet syndrome, acroparaesthesiae.

2 **Peripheral nerve:** peripheral neuritis (diabetic). Nerves involved in general neuropathy are often most vulnerable to pressure, for example, median nerve in the carpal tunnel and ulnar nerve at the elbow(33, 105).

3 **Median nerve** entrapment in the arm (ligament of Struthers)(96), and forearm (pronator teres)(53). Individual branches of the median nerve can be compressed in the hand or digit.

4 **Miscellaneous:** flexor tenosynovitis, myositis, tendinitis.

5 **Functional:** psychoneurosis.

†NB: In patients with carpal tunnel syndrome it is not unusual to find evidence of co-existent cervical spondylosis(68). This may explain the presence of proximal shoulder and neck pain, and the persistence of symptoms after carpal tunnel decompression.

General principles of treatment
Conservative treatment

In patients with mild symptoms the carpal tunnel syndrome often resolves spontaneously.

Conservative treatment – indications

1 Mild symptoms in the absence of abnormal motor signs.
2 In pregnancy where the compression can be expected to subside after delivery.
3 Where there has been an acute or sub-acute connective tissue inflammation, e.g. after Colles' fracture, at the menopause etc.
4 Where the carpal tunnel syndrome has been precipitated by unusual manual labour.

Conservative treatment – types:

1 **Splintage**(38, 102). The carpal tunnel has its maximal capacity when the wrist is splinted in the neutral position or slight extension. Such splintage brings temporary relief to about 70 per cent of patients. A night splint should be used by those who wake at night. A day splint should be used by those who develop symptoms during the day, especially if they have a positive Phalen test.

2 **Restrict hand activity.** When there is a recent onset of symptoms after unusual hand exercise or labour, restrict hand activity. Some patients need to change their occupation.

3 **Corticosteroid injections**(19, 83). Steroid injections into the carpal tunnel may reduce the inflammatory oedema around the median nerve and give temporary relief of symptoms in about 70 per cent of patients.

Rest the patient supine and inject 1.0 ml triamcinolone 10 mg/1 ml with or without local anaesthetic, proximal to the wrist on the ulnar side of the palmaris longus tendon. Use a 25 gauge needle and aim to disperse the solution around the flexor tendons. Inject slowly and take great care to avoid injecting directly into the nerve. Aim the needle distally to enter the carpal tunnel. After injection maintain compression at the injection site, and ask the patient to carry out finger flexion and extension to disperse the steroid.

If no improvement is obtained at the first injection it is unlikely that further injections will help. If improvement is obtained, it is safe to inject two or three more times at weekly or monthly intervals. Relief after steroid injection is a helpful diagnostic point. Some patients experience a transient reactive flare of increased pain.

4 **Drugs.** Diuretics may relieve oedema in pregnancy(110). Oestrogens may be helpful in postmenopausal patients(86). Anti-inflammatory drugs are indicated when there is associated arthritis, epicondylitis, de Quervain's disease.

Vitamin B_6 (pyridoxine hydrochloride) 100 to 200 mg/day for 10 to 12 weeks has been shown to relieve the symptoms of carpal tunnel syndrome where there has not been an associated systemic disease or injury(84).

25
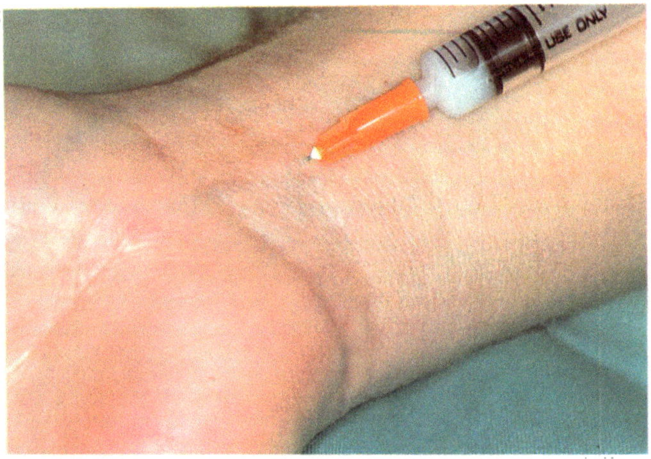

25 Steroid injection of the carpal tunnel. Inject 0.5 ml triamcinolone using a 2 ml syringe and a 25 gauge needle (see page 31).

26a
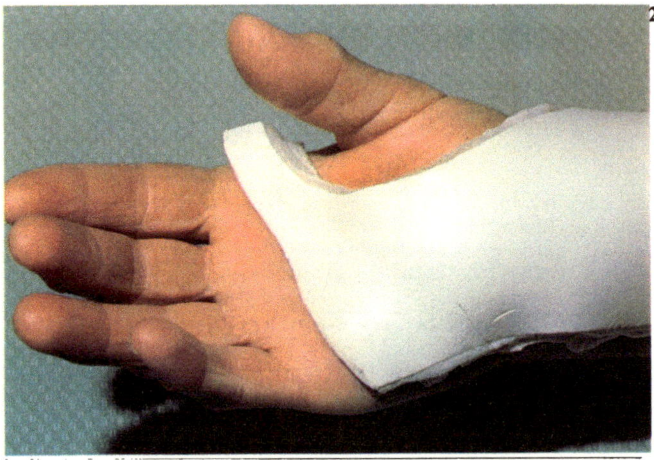

26a A wrist splint is used both as a conservative measure of treatment and, often postoperatively, after removing the sutures.

This splint allows thumb movements and finger movements at the interphalangeal joints. The wrist is in the neutral position or slight extension where the carpal tunnel is at its maximum capacity.

Table 3. Conservative treatment

1	Reduce oedema – diuretic – corticosteroid injection
2	Reduce thickening of flexor tenosynovium – restrict activity
3	Reduce nocturnal wrist flexion – splint

Table 4. Results of conservative treatment (corticosteroid injection and splint)[30]

	Good result	Rate of high relapse
Symptoms	Mild	Severe
Duration	< 1 year	> 1 year
Signs	Normal sensation and motor power	Weakness, muscle atrophy, impaired sensation
EMG	< 2 msec delay in motor and sensory latency	Absent sensory response Motor latency > 6 msec

Operative treatment

Indications

Operative treatment is indicated where there is a specific neurological defect, i.e. compression of the median nerve in the carpal tunnel.

1 Acute carpal tunnel syndrome, with progressive impairment of median nerve function.

2 Chronic carpal tunnel syndrome
(a) Where the symptoms persist despite conservative measures
(b) Signs of impaired sensation, thenar motor weakness or wasting
(c) Evidence of a space-occupying lesion

About 40 per cent of patients require surgical treatment(85).

Warn the patient that his hand:

(a) Will be in a splint and sling for two weeks
(b) Will have restricted use for one month
(c) May be weak for weeks or months
(d) May be painful for a variable time

26b

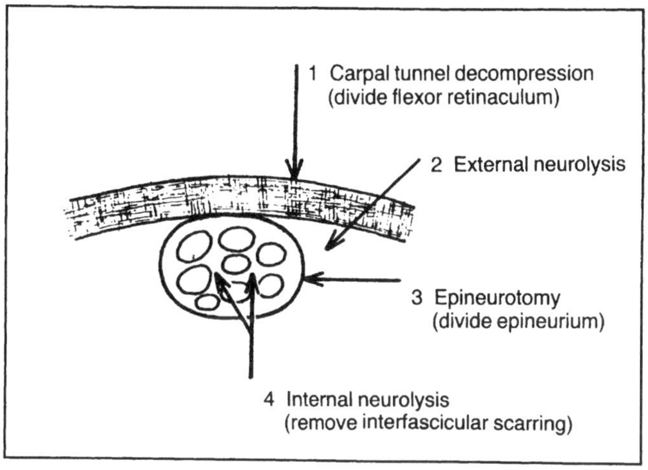

26b Types of operation for median nerve compression. The most common procedure is division of the flexor retinaculum which enlarges the carpal tunnel, so relieving the pressure on the median nerve.

Table 5. Indications for operative treatment

1 Persisting pain. Failed non-operative treatment
2 Objective signs – sensory or motor deficit – space occupying lesion
3 Positive EMG findings?

Table 6. Types of operation according to operative findings of median nerve

Operative finding	Management
Median nerve – normal	Divide flexor retinaculum and related fascia
– congestion	Divide flexor retinaculum and related fascia
– compression	External neurolysis
– epineural fibrosis	Epineurotomy
– intraneural fibrosis	Internal neurolysis
– abnormally large median artery	External neurolysis. Do not resect artery

Treatment of various types of carpal tunnel syndrome

(CTS = carpal tunnel syndrome)
(CTD = carpal tunnel decompression)

1 Conservative treatment	
Minor transient symptoms.	No treatment.
Recent CTS after unusual manual labour.	Restrict hand activity + splint.
Pain at night.	Night splint.
Mild carpal tunnel syndrome, and CTS in pregnancy.	Corticosteroid injection + splint. Diuretics.
2 Operative treatment	
Acute carpal tunnel syndrome (from injury or infection).	Early carpal tunnel decompression (within one to two days)
If symptoms of CTS develop during treatment for acute Colles' fracture.	Loosen bandages and cast. Extend wrist to neutral position.
If tardy median palsy develops after Colles' fracture.	CTD. (After Colles' fracture CTS can occur within hours, months, or years after injury. It commonly occurs within three months.)
Persisting carpal tunnel syndrome (with thenar muscle signs or impaired sensation):	Elective carpal tunnel decompression.
(a) Median nerve compressed by rheumatoid proliferative flexor tenosynovium.	Partial flexor tenosynovectomy.
(b) Proliferative flexor tenosynovium and incipient flexor tendon rupture.	Complete flexor tenosynovectomy.
(c) Median nerve constricted by fibrosis (external or internal).	Median neurolysis (external neurolysis, epineurotomy or internal neurolysis).
(d) Thenar muscle palsy with lack of opposition.	Consider opposition tendon transfer.
(e) Space-occupying lesion, for example, ganglion.	Neurolysis and resect space-occupying lesion.
Pressure from a large patent median artery.	Do not resect the median artery[62].
Bilateral carpal tunnel syndrome.	CTD on the worst-affected hand. Treat less-involved hand by conservative measures. Do not decompress both hands at the one time.
Co-existent Dupuytren's disease.	Avoid performing fasciectomy at the same time as carpal tunnel decompression.
Co-existent Raynaud's phenomenon.	CTD (vascular improvement may be incomplete).
Persistent carpal tunnel syndrome, after operation.	Re-operate. Divide the flexor retinaculum and its proximal and distal fascial attachments. Perform external and internal neurolysis as necessary.
Recurrent carpal tunnel syndrome.	Re-operate as above.

Postoperative treatment

Aim to prevent swelling and stiffness by maintaining wrist splintage, hand and arm elevation, and finger exercises.

Postoperative period	**Management**
Days one and two	Keep the patient in hospital with hand and arm elevated, until any postoperative pain and swelling has subsided. Begin active finger movements.
Weeks one and two	Splint the wrist for two weeks. Avoid dependency. When a sling is worn the patient is told to remove the sling several times daily, and to exercise the elbow and shoulder through a full range of movement.
Weeks three and four	Maintain a firm bandage support of the wrist. Allow only light activities.
Weeks five to eight	Should be able to resume most forms of light work. Avoid heavy gripping or repetitive work for about three months.

Complications[18, 22, 42, 58, 72, 93]

Carpal tunnel decompression may be associated with one or more of the following complications (in about 10 per cent of patients[72]).

Intraoperative

1 Iatrogenic injury to:
- median nerve trunk
- palmar branch*
- recurrent thenar branch
- digital branches

2 Inadequate carpal tunnel decompression from inadequate division of the flexor retinaculum.

Postoperative

1 Early
- haematoma (from damage to the superficial palmar arch)
- oedema
- wound complications (infection and dehiscence have occurred in those patients treated preoperatively by corticosteroid injection)

2 Later
- weakness of grip (may last months)
- stiffness of the fingers, wrist, and shoulder†
- pain (in the wound from cutaneous nerve entrapped in scar (see **47**), in the retracted edges of the flexor retinaculum, and in the wrist from loss of carpal support)
- scar hypertrophy and contracture from incision perpendicular to the wrist crease
- palmar fasciitis
- sympathetic dystrophy[72] (causalgia all too frequently results from minor trauma to the median nerve)

3 Recurrent carpal tunnel syndrome from fibrosis around the median nerve or hyperplasia of the tenosynovium

4 Other complications
- bowstringing of the flexor tendons
- adhesions of the flexor tendons after flexor tenosynovectomy

*Neuroma of the palmar branch can lead to disability far greater than the original disorder of carpal tunnel syndrome.

†Stiffness of the non-operated parts of the hand from pain, swelling or scar can be more disabling than the original sensory signs[70].

Table 7. Postoperative complications

Early	Haematoma Pain Swelling and stiffness
Later	Median neuritis Fibrosis of carpal tunnel contents Recurrent carpal tunnel syndrome

Table 8. Four keys to successful surgical technique

1 Basic hand surgical principles (bloodless field, loupe magnification)
2 Adequate decompression of the flexor retinaculum and related fascial structures
3 Adequate exposure of the median nerve and its terminal branches
4 Avoid unnecessary handling and exploration of structures which are not directly involved in the compressive syndrome

Results of carpal tunnel decompression[20, 42, 93]

Surgical release of the flexor retinaculum and its proximal and distal fascial attachments, with or without external or internal neurolysis, usually eliminates compression of the median nerve, with relief of most of the symptoms of carpal tunnel syndrome in about 85 per cent of patients, provided there has been no degeneration of nerve endings[93].

The relief of pain is usually prompt if the carpal tunnel decompression is carried out within 6 months of the onset of symptoms. The recovery of sensory impairment is less likely to be prompt[82]. Weakness and wasting is usually more delayed in recovery[20]. Though established severe muscle wasting may not recover, moderate thenar atrophy often is reversible.

Success or failure in relieving the symptoms and signs of carpal tunnel syndrome depends on:

1 Motivation of the patient
2 Judgement and skills of the operating surgeon
3 Duration of the carpal tunnel syndrome and
4 The type of pathology in the carpal tunnel and the median nerve.

The best results follow in a well motivated patient who has had definite clinical features of a carpal tunnel syndrome for six months or less and who at operation is found to have a mildly congested median nerve.

Many patients whose carpal tunnel syndrome is associated with occupational flexor tenosynovitis have residual pain of ill-defined nature for many months after operation. For this reason one should be cautious in selection for surgery and not promise relief of all symptoms.

If a patient has had adequate carpal tunnel decompression and median neurolysis (external or internal) and has not had a significant release of symptoms, the diagnosis is in doubt and the prognosis guarded. It is unwise to re-operate unless some new condition has developed. For indications for re-operation see page 73.

In about 10 per cent of patients there are poor results, possibly from chronic changes (demyelination) in the median nerve itself. In one series 9 per cent of patients were not improved or were actually worse postoperatively. Neither inadequate surgery nor incorrect diagnosis were held responsible[20].

It is rare to have disability from division of the flexor retinaculum although postoperative widening of the carpal arch has been observed. Bowstringing is a rare complication[72].

Table 9a. Results of carpal tunnel decompression*

Relief of	Pain[93]	Immediate
	Numbness[20, 42]	Slow and ? incomplete
	Weakness and wasting[20, 42]	Slow and ? incomplete
	Delay in nerve conductivity[35, 36, 40]	Improves slowly (1 to 2 years)

*If done within 6 months of onset of symptoms and before degeneration of nerve endings.

Table 9b. Results of carpal tunnel decompression[20]

Very good	Total relief of symptoms	50%
Good	75% or greater improvement	30%
Fair	50% or greater improvement	10%
Poor	No improvement or worse	10%

27

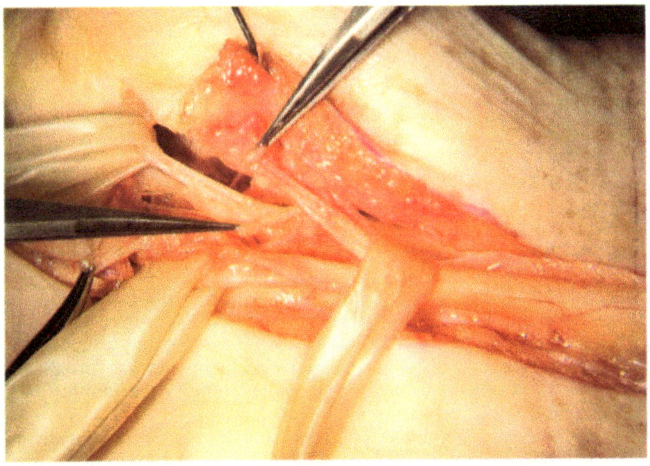

28

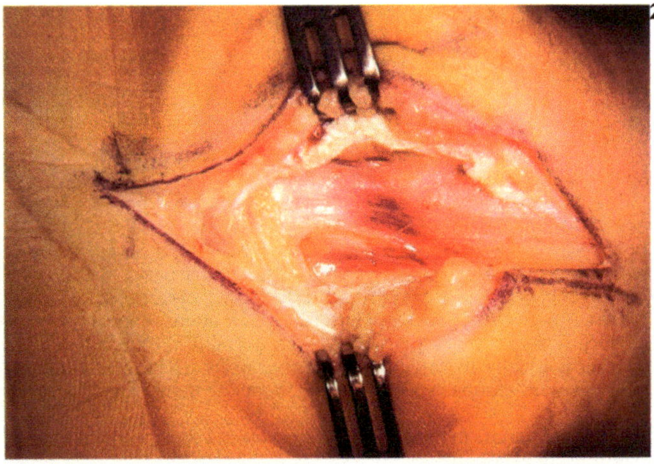

29

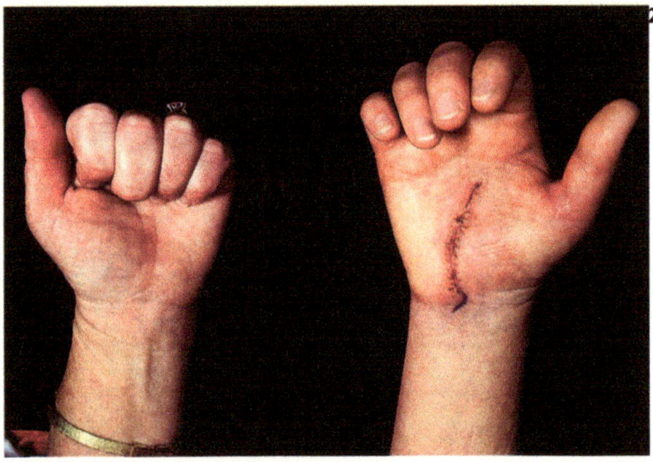

27 Iatrogenic division of the median nerve. Persistent numbness and weakness after carpal tunnel decompression.

Four months ago this 30-year-old labourer had right carpal tunnel decompression through a transverse wrist incision. 'Blind' section of the flexor retinaculum resulted in accidental division of the radial part of the median nerve. The two cut ends of the nerve are held in micro-forceps.

28 Inadequate carpal tunnel decompression. Persisting carpal tunnel syndrome six months after carpal tunnel decompression. Only the proximal half of the flexor retinaculum had been divided through a short oblique wrist incision.

Operative findings. Severe congestion of the median nerve.

29 Postoperative swelling, stiffness, and early palmar fasciitis. Three days after operation this 40-year-old secretary developed pain which persisted for three months. She developed a sympathetic dystrophy.

Part B Carpal tunnel decompression (and related procedures) – surgical techniques

Contents

Surgical anatomy of the median nerve

30a

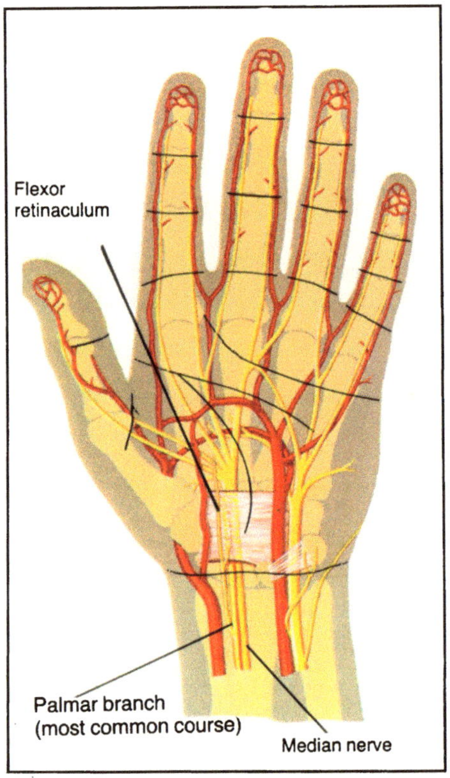

30b

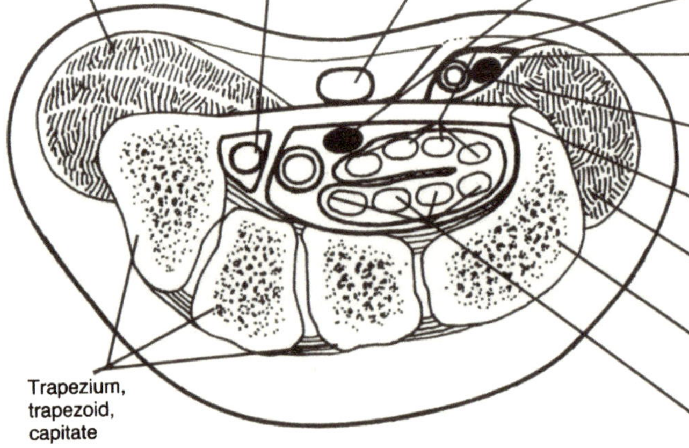

30a Diagram of nerves and vessels of the hand in relation to bones, flexor retinaculum and skin markings. Note the distal volar skin crease of the wrist represents the proximal border of the flexor retinaculum, which extends about 3 cm distal to that crease.

30b Cross section of the carpal tunnel.

Anatomical variations of the median nerve in the carpal tunnel were found in 29 of 246 hands explored at operation(60).

Variations may be classified into four groups:
1 Variation in the course of the recurrent thenar motor branch (extra ligamentous 46 per cent, subligamentous 31 per cent, and trans-ligamentous 23 per cent).
2 Accessory branches at the distal portion of the carpal tunnel.
3 High division of the median nerve and
4 Accessory branches proximal to the carpal tunnel.

Branches may arise from the ulnar side of the median nerve, not only distal to the carpal tunnel but also within or proximal to it. Thus, it is safer to approach the median nerve from the ulnar side when opening the carpal tunnel.

31

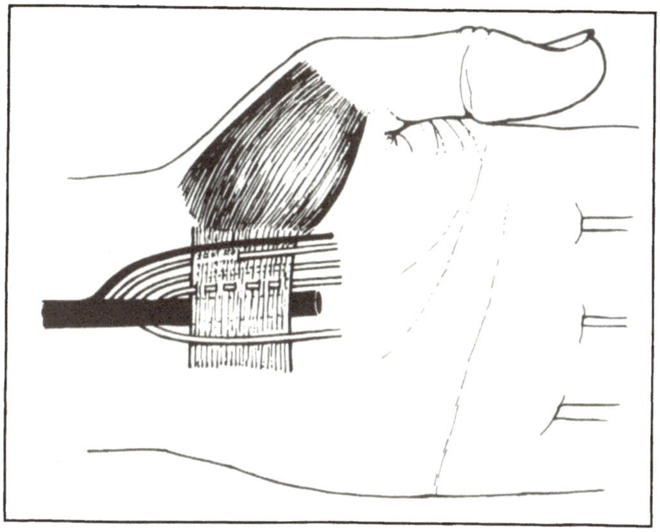

31 Palmar branch. Variations in anatomy. The palmar branch arises usually from the radial aspect of the median nerve as it emerges from the radial margin of the flexor digitorum superficialis, usually 5 cm proximal to the radial styloid. It separates from the nerve trunk but runs parallel to it along its radial border to a point 1 cm proximal to the flexor retinaculum where it passes through its own tunnel within the flexor retinaculum just ulnar to the flexor carpi radialis. There it divides into its terminal branches. These pass through the palmar fascia to supply a variable degree of skin overlying the thenar eminence at the base of the palm.

32

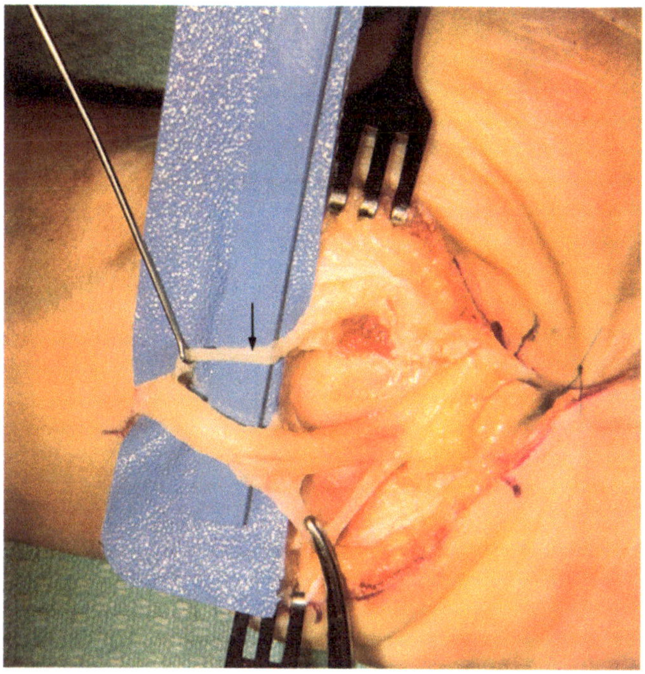

32 Palmar branch of the median nerve (arrow) penetrating the flexor retinaculum.

33

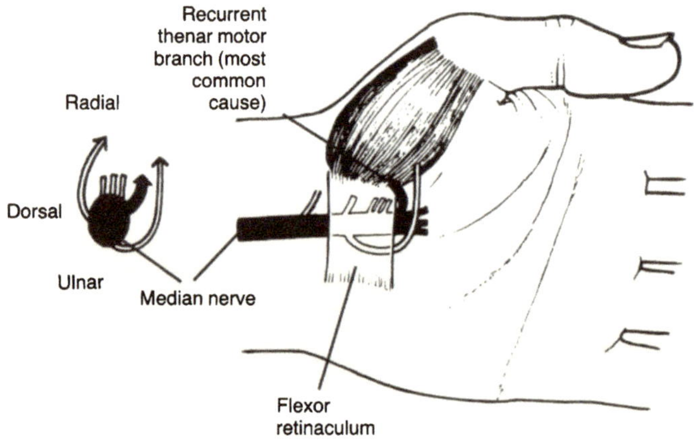

33 Recurrent thenar motor branch. Variations in anatomy. The recurrent thenar motor branch usually arises as a single branch from the radial side of the median nerve just distal to the retinaculum. It recurs back over the retinaculum into the thenar muscles.

It may also arise at more proximal levels, from the volar, ulnar or dorsal aspect of the median nerve. It may run superficial or deep to the flexor retinaculum.

The recurrent thenar motor branch can be absent and the thenar muscles all supplied by the ulnar nerve. Aberrant thenar muscles, e.g. enlargement of the superficial head of the flexor pollicis brevis may be a clue to an aberrant thenar muscle branch(100).

34

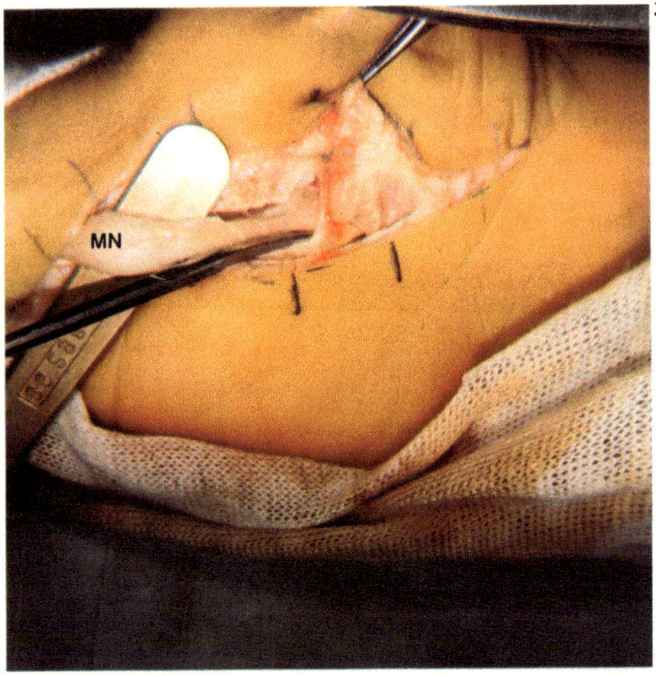

34 The recurrent thenar motor branch arising from the ulnar aspect of the median nerve (MN) and coursing volar across the nerve to the thenar muscles – left hand.

35

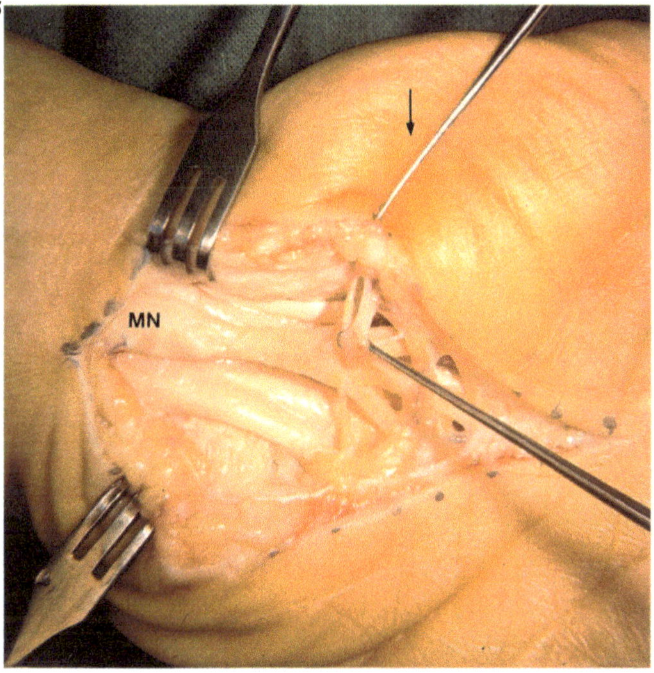

36

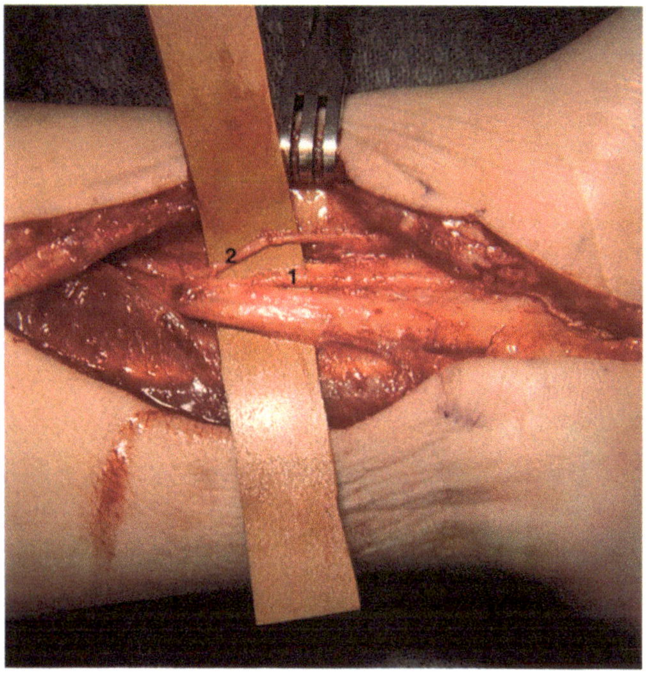

35 Two recurrent thenar branches arising from the volar aspect of the left median nerve (MN). Note the thenar muscle wasting (arrowed).

36 High origin of the recurrent thenar branch (1) arising 1 cm distal to the palmar branch (2).

Abnormal contents of the carpal tunnel

37

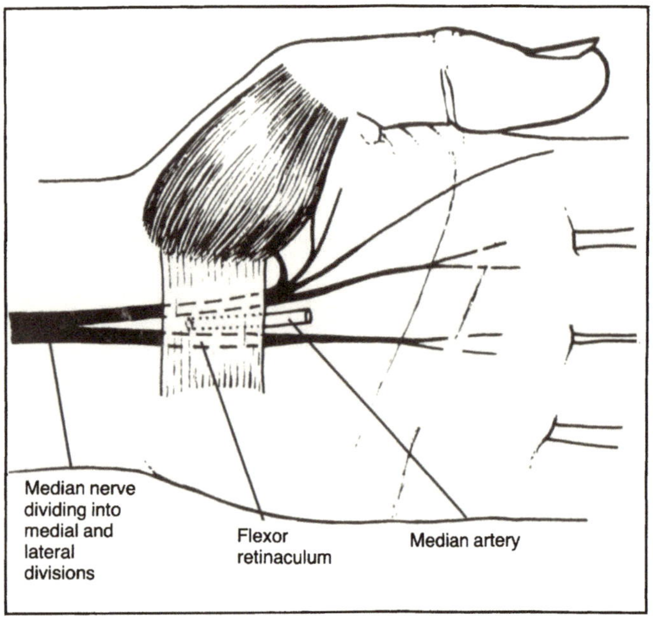

37 The median nerve trunk. High division of the trunk into medial and lateral divisions in the low forearm. A persistent median artery often lies between the two divisions. Rarely this artery can thrombose and cause CTS(12).

Caution – when you have found the median nerve, look for another.

38

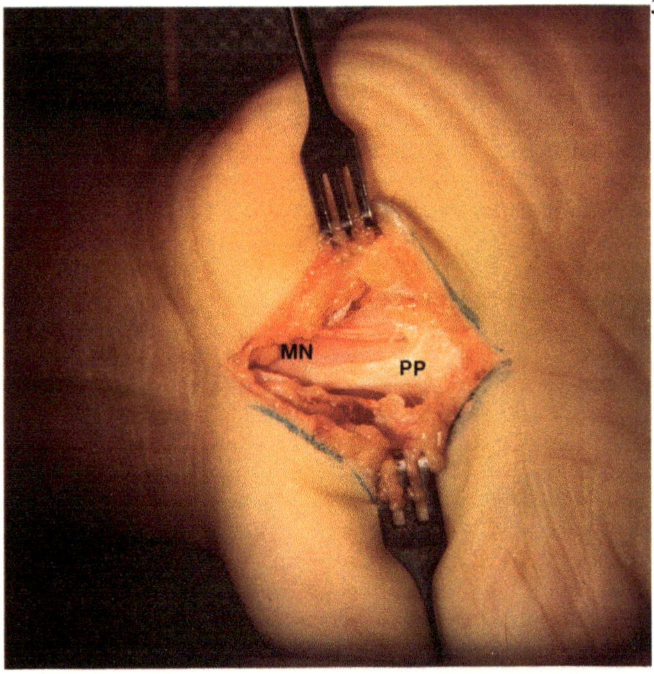

38 Palmaris profundus (PP) presenting as the most superficial structure in the carpal tunnel. The median nerve (MN) is partly obscured.

Preoperative management for carpal tunnel decompression

1 Routine hand measures

(a) The patient: He/she should stop smoking, have a general medical check (urine, blood pressure, etc.), and be asked about medications and allergies.

(b) The hand: Remove rings, jewellery, and nail varnish. Trim the fingernails.

2 Specific for carpal tunnel decompression

Check for an underlying cause, for example, rheumatoid arthritis, flexor tenosynovitis, Raynaud's condition, space-occupying lesion, etc.

Anaesthesia

A **brachial plexus or axillary nerve block** provides optimal operative and postoperative conditions. The hand remains painless and paralysed for some hours. The patient and the nursing staff can concentrate on maintaining elevation of the hand, reducing the chance of postoperative bleeding.

Any nerve block – brachial, axillary or wrist – may be complicated by neuritis, which may cause pain and discomfort for several weeks or months. Therefore, such nerve blocks are unwise in those who use their hands for fine work, for example, musicians, artists, and surgeons. In these people and in those who are nervous or apprehensive and more prone to neuritis complications, a general anaesthetic is preferred.

Occasionally a brachial plexus nerve block is complicated by a pneumothorax.

Local anaesthesia allows the surgeon to assess the effect of active finger movement on the dynamics of the carpal tunnel. A lumbrical muscle with an abnormally high origin can increase the contents of the carpal tunnel during active finger flexion and so produce median nerve compression[40].

A **Bier's regional anaesthetic** is also used.

39

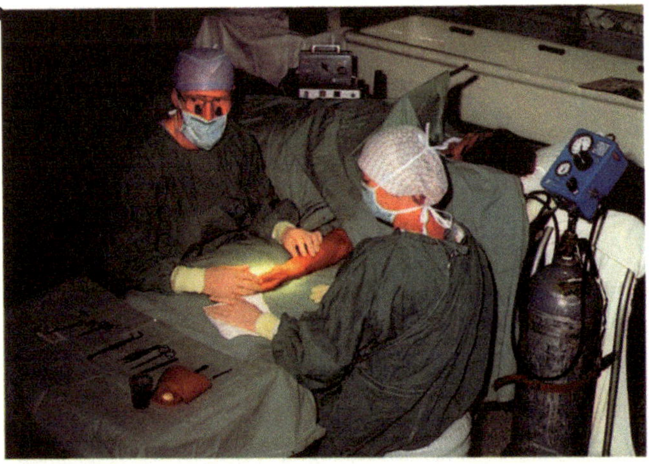

40

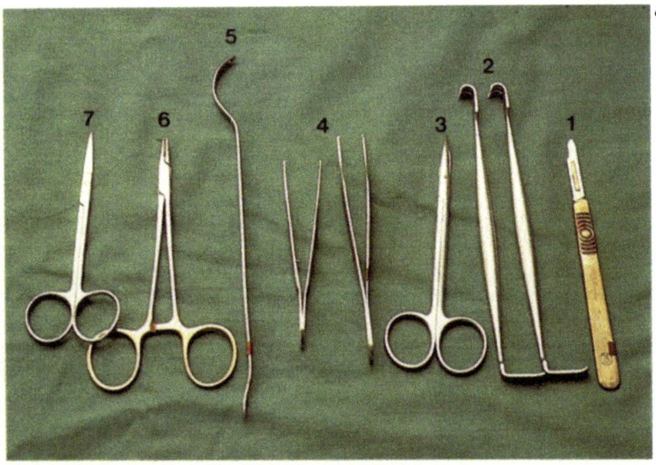

41

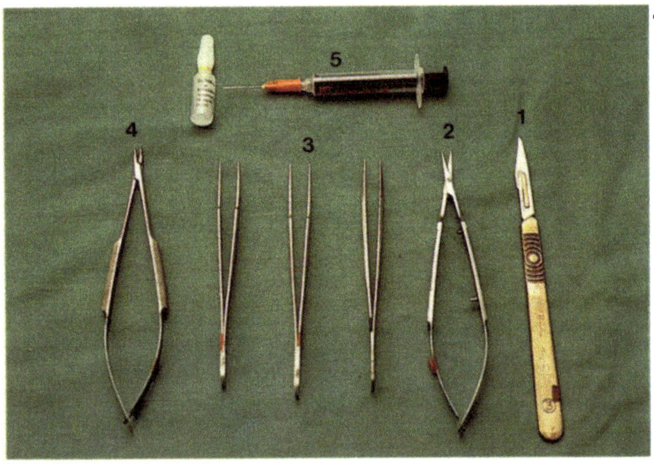

39 The hand operation. Note that –
1 The patient has had regional anaesthetic.
2 The surgeon operates with the aid of a magnifying loupe. This is essential if the surgeon is to dissect safely the median nerve and its branches.
3 The pneumatic tourniquet is an essential adjunct in hand surgery. The precise anatomical dissection essential in hand surgical procedures requires a quiet, bloodless field.

40 Routine instruments for carpal tunnel decompression. (1) Scalpel with size 15 blade; (2) rake retractors; (3) dissecting scissors; (4) fine-toothed dissecting forceps; (5) dissector; (6) needle holder, and (7) suture-cutting scissors.

41 Microsurgical instruments for internal neurolysis. (1) Scalpel with No. 11 or beaver blade; (2) micro-scissors; (3) jeweller's forceps; (4) micro-needle holder; (5) 2 ml syringe and triamcinolone suspension.

Incision

42

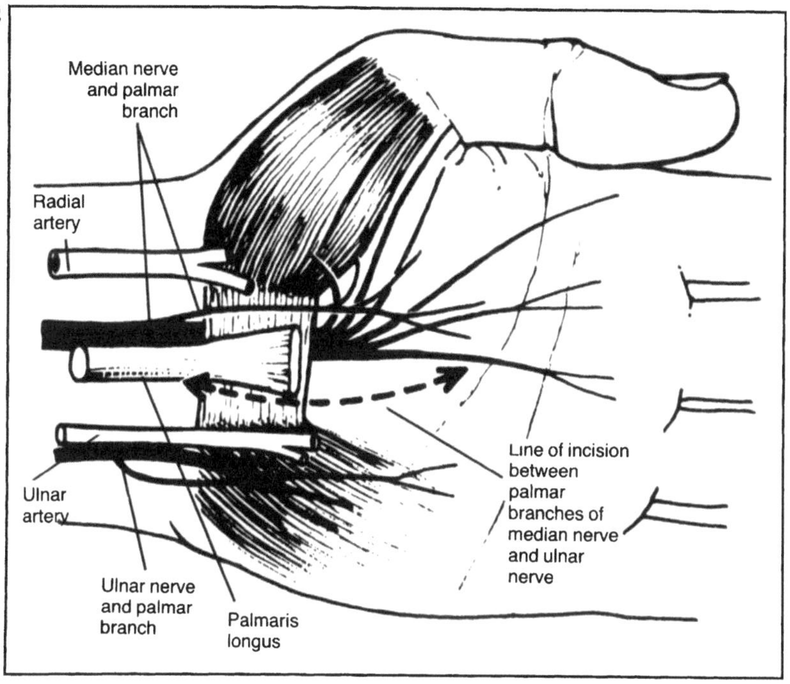

42 Skin incision. This is made on the ulnar side of the thenar crease, between the palmar branches of the median and ulnar nerves. A vertical line bisecting the ring finger approximates the boundary between these two nerves. This incision avoids all but a few terminal branches of these nerves.

The palmar branch of the median nerve lies between the palmaris longus and flexor carpi radialis tendons at the wrist.

Accidental division of the palmar branch of the median nerve can lead to a sensitive neuroma in the scar.

Caution – 'Blind' carpal tunnel decompression through a transverse incision is dangerous and may result in:

1 Cutting the median nerve or its branches.

2 Incomplete division of the flexor retinaculum with persisting symptoms and signs (see page 73). Blind section makes inspection of the carpal tunnel impossible(42).

43
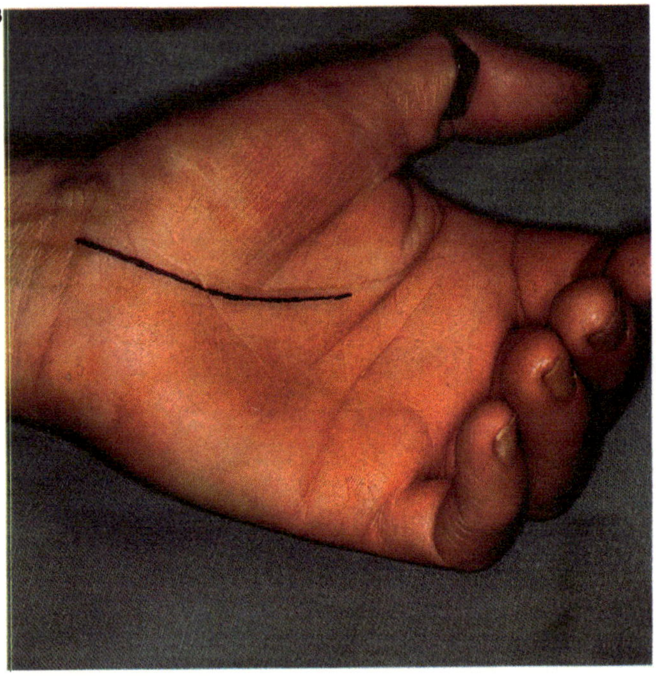

44
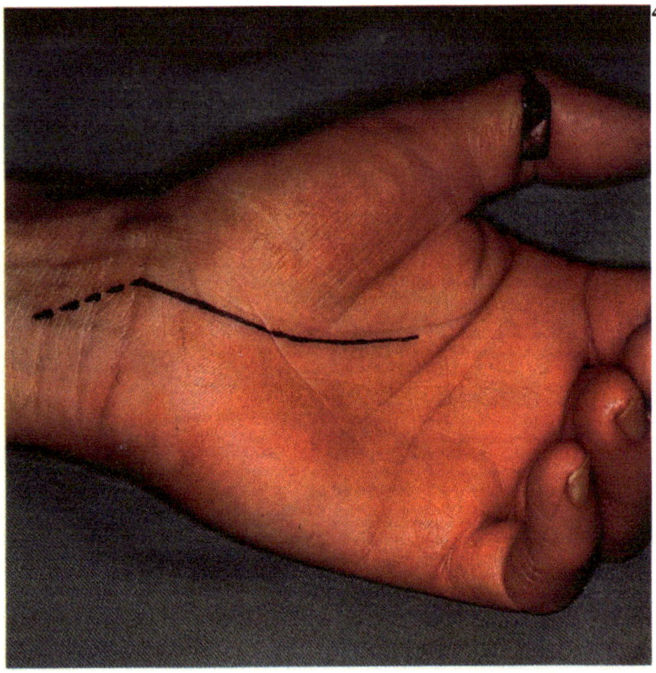

43 Mark the incision parallel to and on the ulnar side of the thenar crease (linea vitalis)*, from the level of the tip of the outstretched thumb to the distal wrist crease.

These levels correspond to the level of the superficial palmar arch and the proximal edge of the flexor retinaculum (see **30a**).

*Linea vitalis = 'life line'.

44 Exposure proximal to the wrist crease into the distal forearm may be necessary for:

1 Relief of median nerve compression by the volar carpal ligament or the deep fascia of the forearm.

2 Flexor tenosynovectomy.

Such an extension should be made obliquely at an angle of about 45° in an ulnar direction into the distal forearm, to avoid scar contracture across the wrist crease.

45

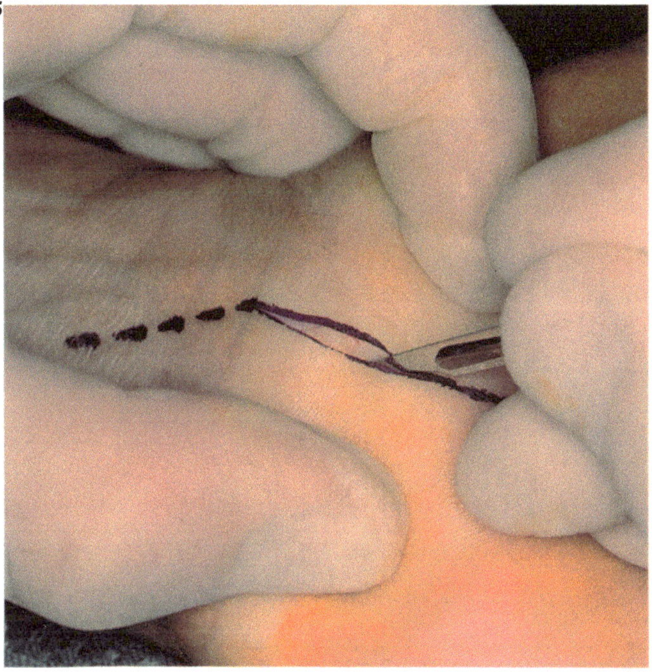

45 Making the incision. Use a scalpel with a size 15 blade. For maximal control hold the scalpel near the blade.

Support the tissues adjacent to the wound using thumb and index finger.

46

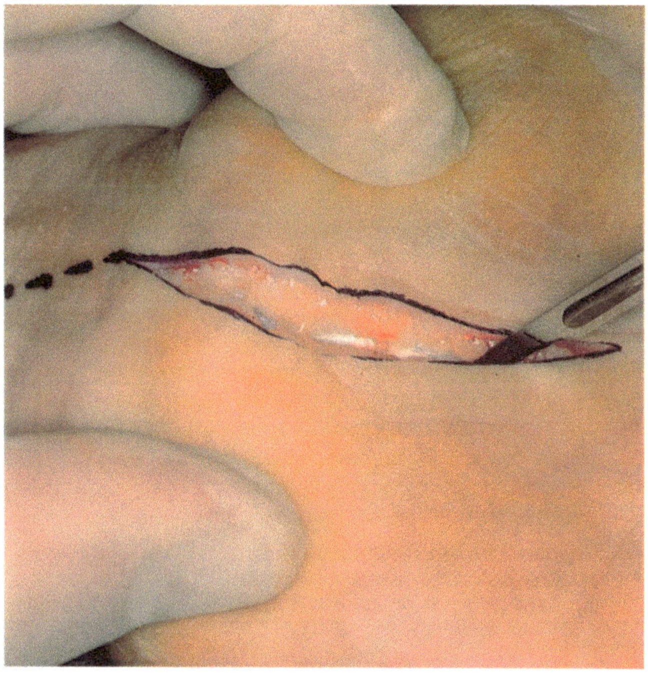

46 Incise vertically through the skin and subcutaneous fat to the level of the palmar aponeurosis.

Minimise the dissection of skin and subcutaneous tissues, especially on the radial side. Palmar branches of the median nerve sometimes enter the overlying skin through the flexor retinaculum itself, and this portion of the skin flap will be denervated and a neuroma might develop if those branches are cut.

Caution – The making of the incision and exposure is most important. As many as one-third of patients may have long-lasting discomfort in the operative scar[20].

Exposure

47

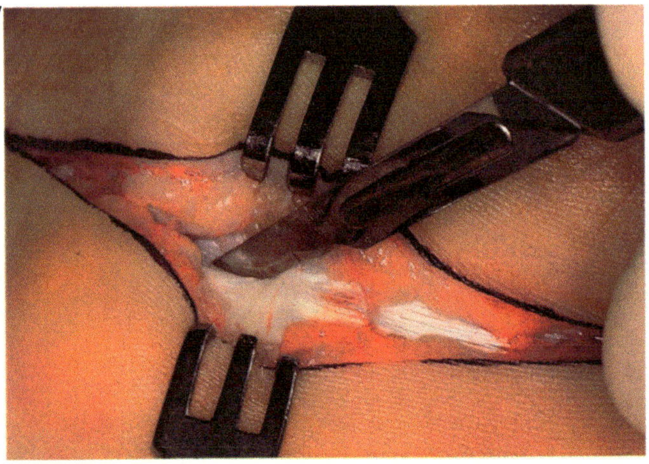

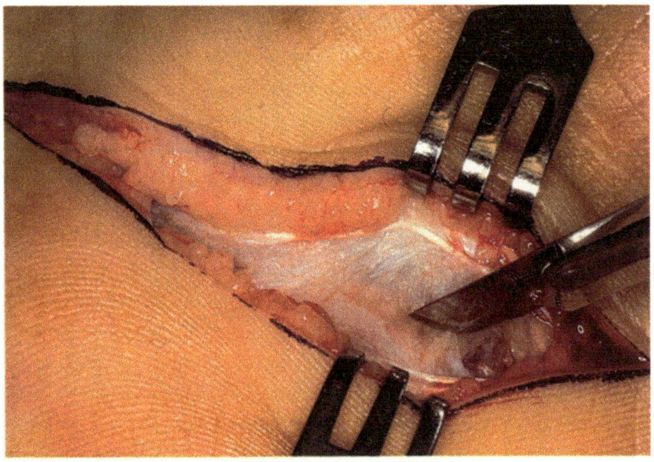

47 Exposure. Use rake retractors to retract the skin and subcutaneous tissues and so display the palmar aponeurosis.

Large blood vessels in this plane may occasionally need fine ligature (4/0 or 5/0 catgut) or coagulation (preferably bipolar or at least fine point coagulation).

Caution – Avoid the palmar branch of the median nerve. Wear a magnifying loupe to aid in the safe dissection of the median nerve and its branches.

If the palmar branch is cut, dissect it proximally and section it at its origin from the median nerve.

Do not attempt to repair the palmar branch, because a disabling neuroma will probably develop.

48 Incise the palmar aponeurosis.

Caution – Do not mistake this layer for the flexor retinaculum itself. The superficial fibres of the palmar aponeurosis are longitudinal, the deeper ones run irregularly and obliquely. The fibres of the flexor retinaculum run transversely.

Expose the fatty tissue distal to the flexor retinaculum around the superficial palmar vessels.

The flexor retinaculum can extend 3 to 4 cm distal to the distal volar crease of the wrist, and can present here as a thinned out layer which may be mistaken for the mid-palmar fascia(88)*. The thenar motor recurrent branch is vulnerable at this point.*

49

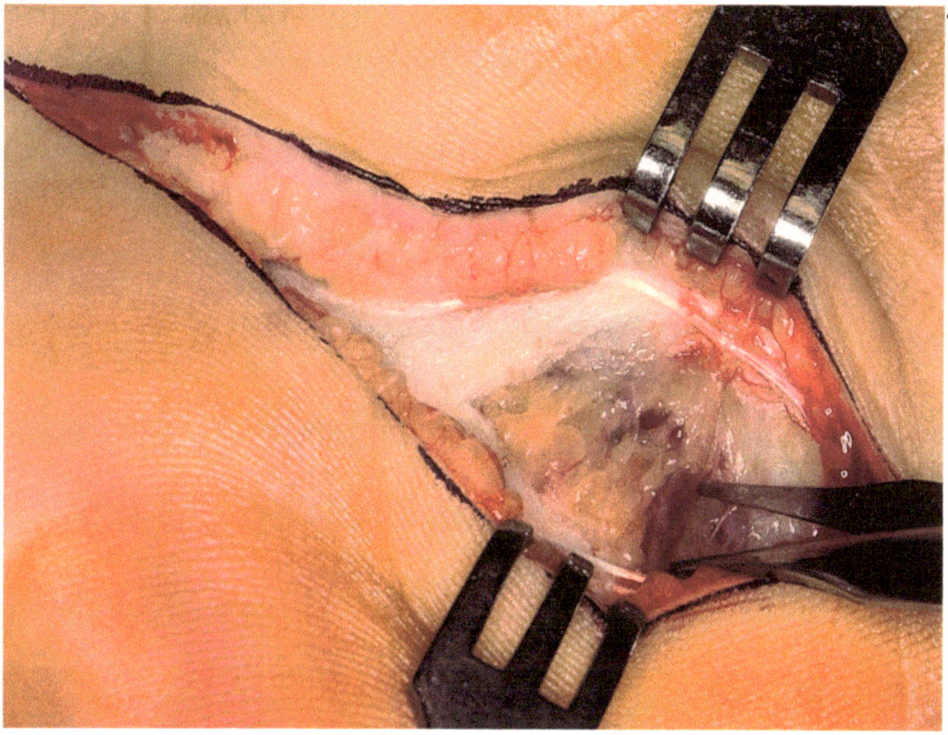

49 Superficial palmar arch. With scalpel or scissors expose the superficial palmar arch. This should be the distal limit of dissection, because any nerve compression will be proximal to this point.

The distal edge of the flexor retinaculum is about 1 cm proximal to the arch.

Division of the flexor retinaculum and related fascia

50a

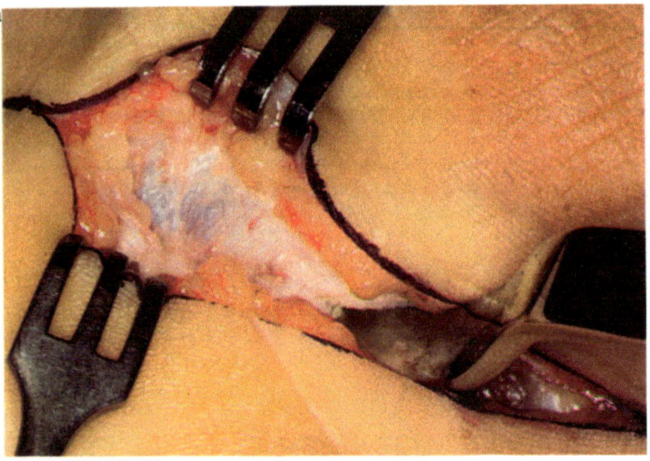

50a Flexor retinaculum. Expose the distal part of the flexor retinaculum which is at a deep level. The retinaculum slants dorsally and does not lie parallel to the plane of the hand.

Protect the median nerve, which lies to the radial side of the midline and in close contact with the deep surface of the retinaculum. Pass a moistened dissector or haemostat gently, with fingertip control, beneath the distal edge of the flexor retinaculum to separate the median nerve and flexor tendon structures from the deep surface of the retinaculum.

Beware of variations in the anatomy of the median nerve (page 40). Do not pass the dissector deep to an anomalous recurrent thenar motor branch[41].

50b

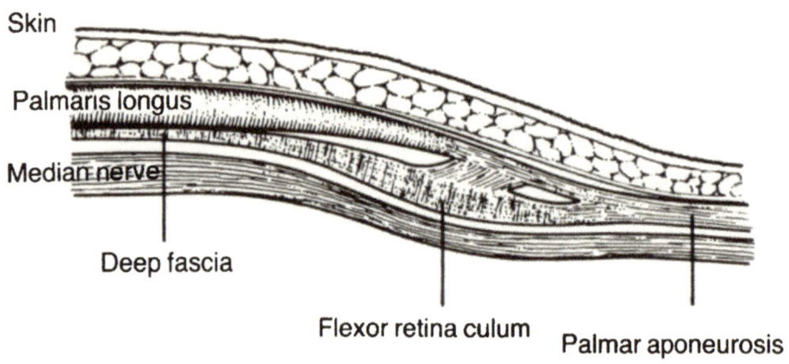

50b Fascial relations of the flexor retinaculum and the median nerve. The median nerve is mostly compressed at the distal part of the flexor retinaculum, which is deeper and thicker and more distal than is often appreciated.

51

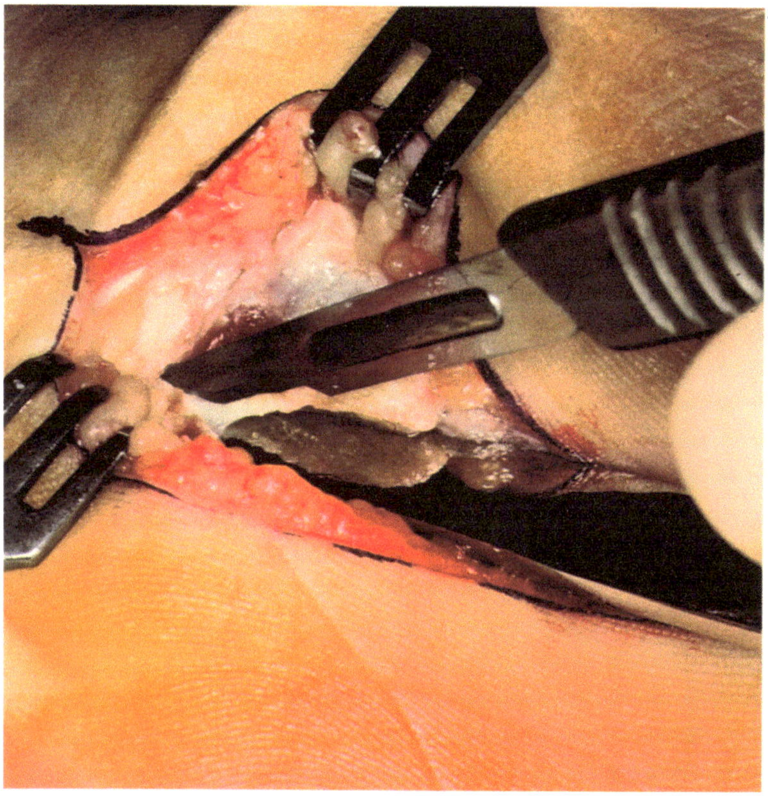

51 Incise the flexor retinaculum on the ulnar side of the midline to avoid damage to the median nerve or its thenar motor branch. Anatomical variations of the median nerve in the carpal tunnel are found in 10 per cent of cases(60).

Muscle fibres of the thenar and hypothenar group are often seen arising from the radial and ulnar side of the flexor retinaculum.

Caution – Be on the lookout for an aberrant palmar branch of the median nerve or an aberrant recurrent thenar motor branch. Anomalous attachments of the thenar muscles to the distal part of the flexor retinaculum would suggest such an aberrant recurrent thenar motor branch to those muscles.

A recurrent thenar branch will usually recur around the distal edge of the flexor retinaculum, but it may perforate the distal border of the ligament.

52a

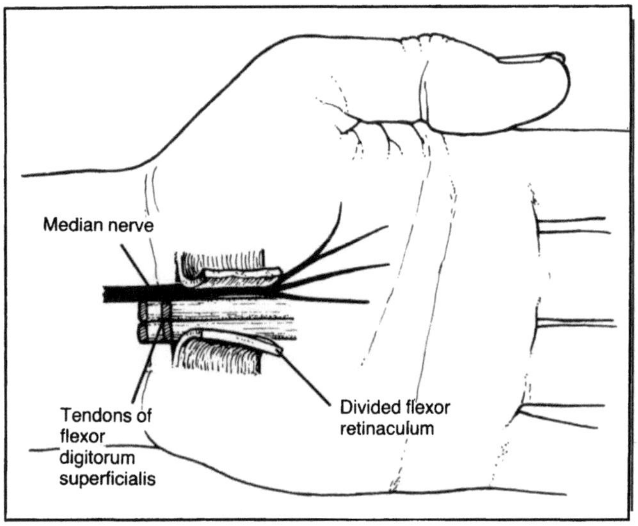

52b

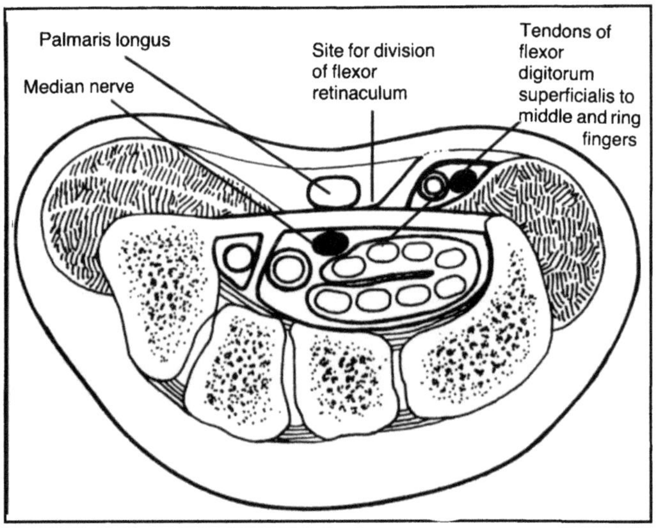

52a Incise the flexor retinaculum on the ulnar side of the midline. This should expose the flexor superficialis tendons. The median nerve should lie beneath the radial part of the flexor retinaculum.

52b Site for division of the flexor retinaculum. Approach the median nerve from the ulnar side.

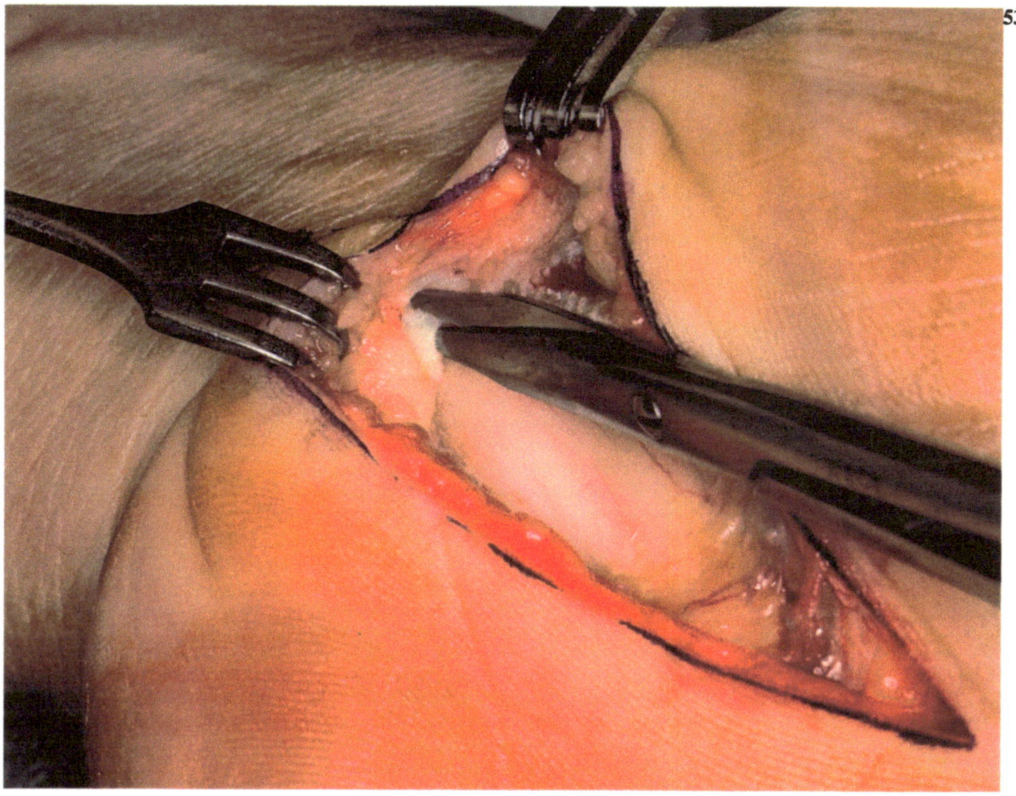

53

53 Retract the edges of the proximal part of the wound and using fine blunt-nosed dissecting scissors, again under direct vision, cut the proximal part of the flexor retinaculum on the ulnar side of the median nerve.

Check that all fibres of the flexor retinaculum have been divided. Any fibres not sectioned can be responsible for persistent median nerve compression. It is not necessary to biopsy or resect part of the retinaculum.

There is a considerable amount of subcutaneous fat at the bases of the thenar and hypothenar eminences which will need to be retracted to show the retinaculum.

Incomplete division of the flexor retinaculum is the commonest cause of failure of the operation.

54

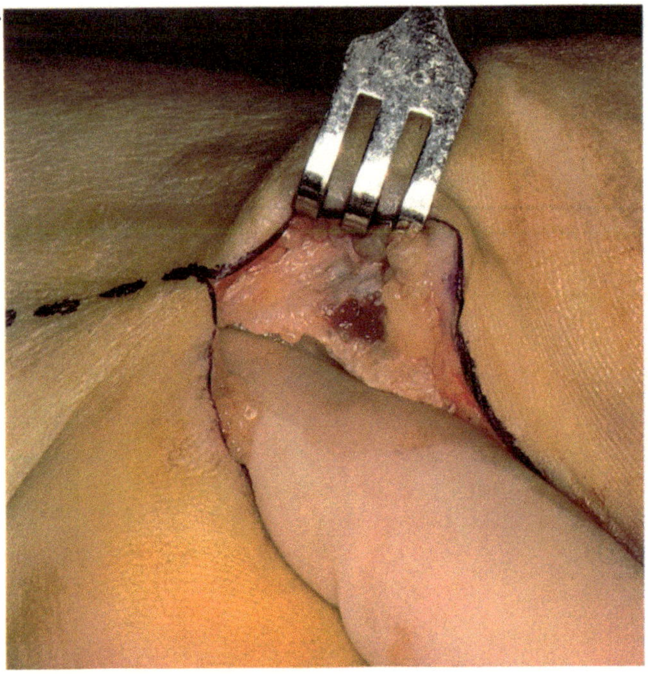

54 Proximal decompression. Now exclude compression of the median nerve proximal to the carpal tunnel.

Pass your little or index finger between the divided parts of the flexor retinaculum in the proximal part of the wound up the forearm, to check that the deep fascia of the forearm is not compressing the median nerve.

55

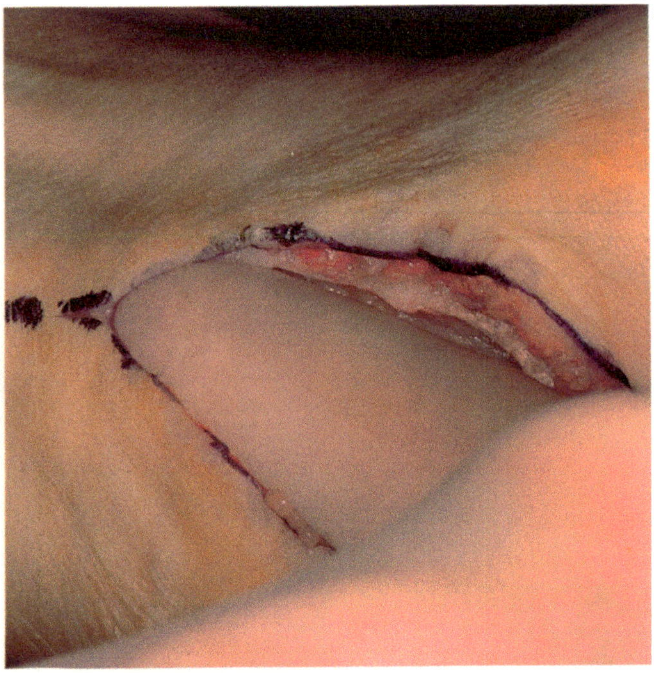

55 If the finger does not pass freely, divide the distal deep fascia of the forearm for about 3 cm. It may be necessary, as it was in this case, to extend the skin incision above the wrist.

56

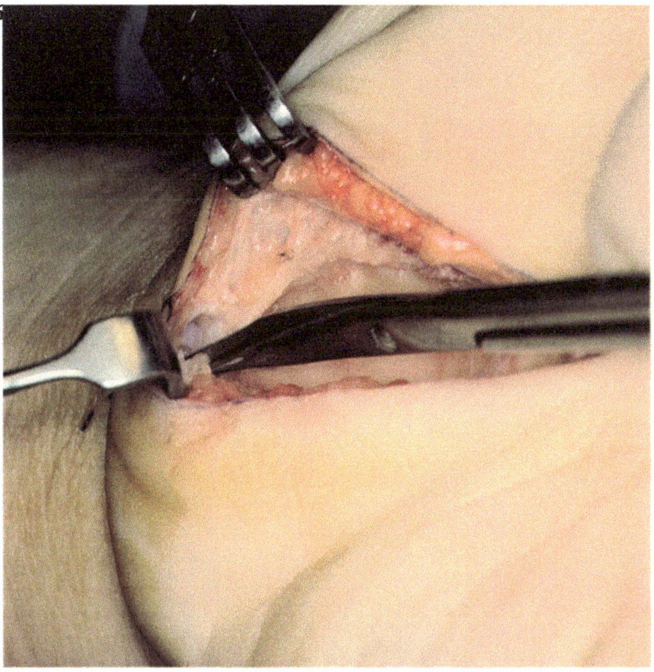

57

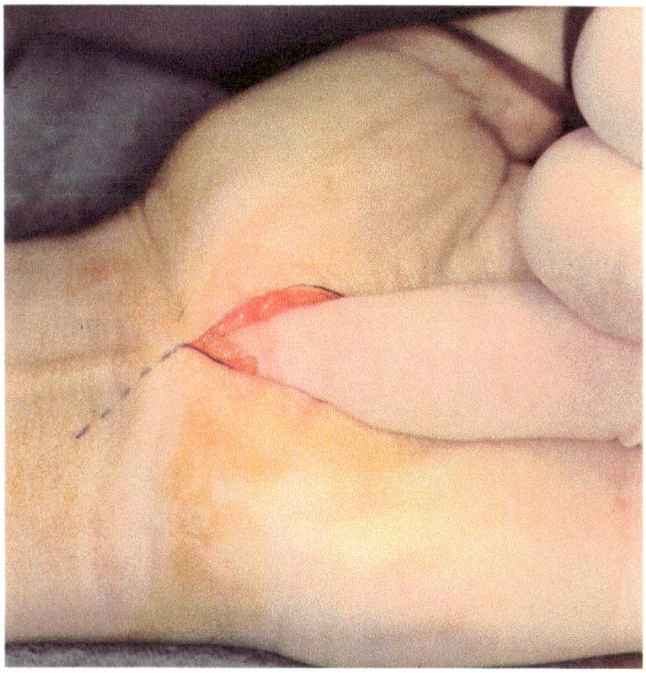

56 and 57 Division of proximal part of the flexor retinaculum. In this operation on another patient the proximal part of the flexor retinaculum was divided. The deep fascia of the forearm, however, obstructed free passage of the little finger proximal to the wrist.

58
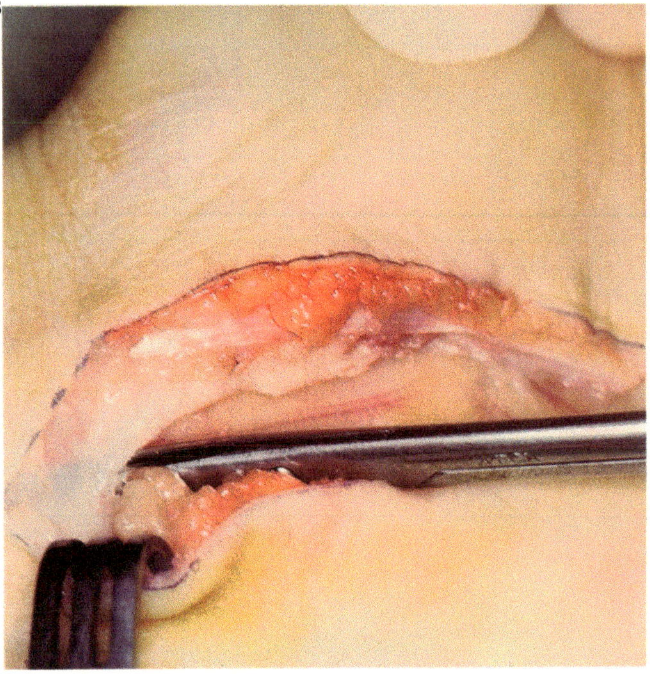

59
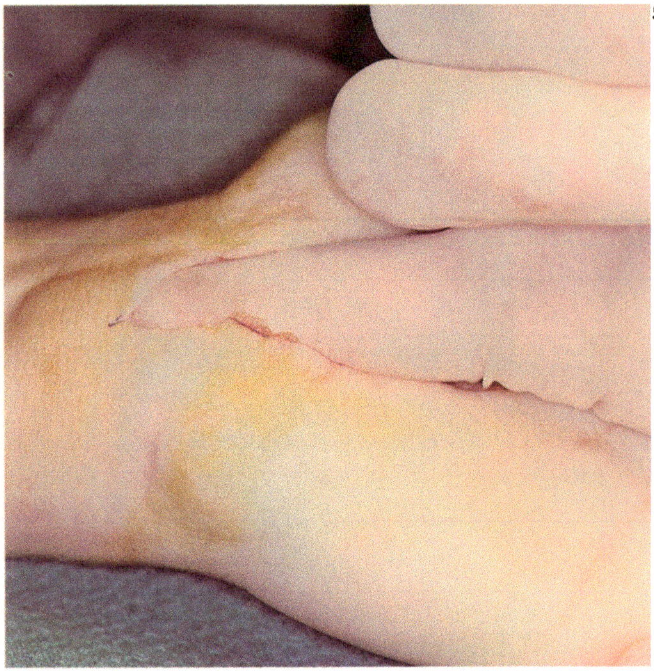

58 and 59 Incision of the skin and that deep fascia continuous with the proximal part of the flexor retinaculum then allowed free passage of the finger, thus ensuring absence of compression of the median nerve as it passes from the forearm into the carpal tunnel.

60

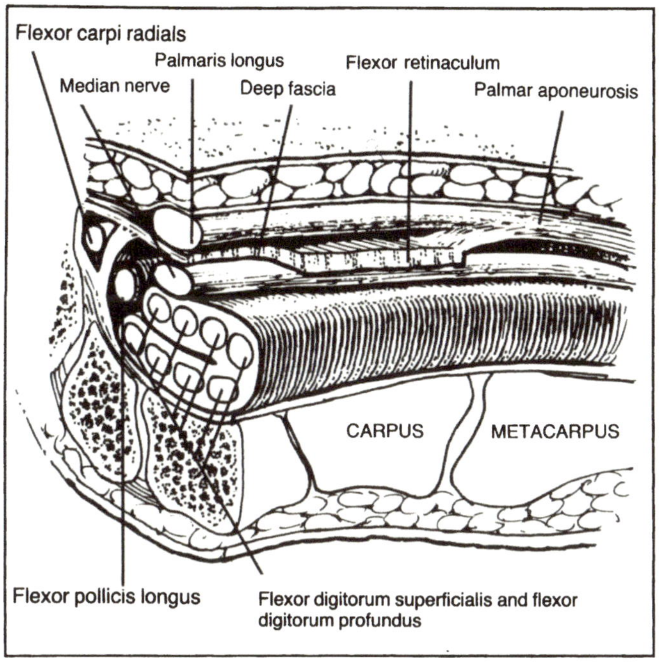

60 Diagram of the fascial relations of the flexor retinaculum. The obliquity of the flexor retinaculum is not shown in this diagram (see **51b**).

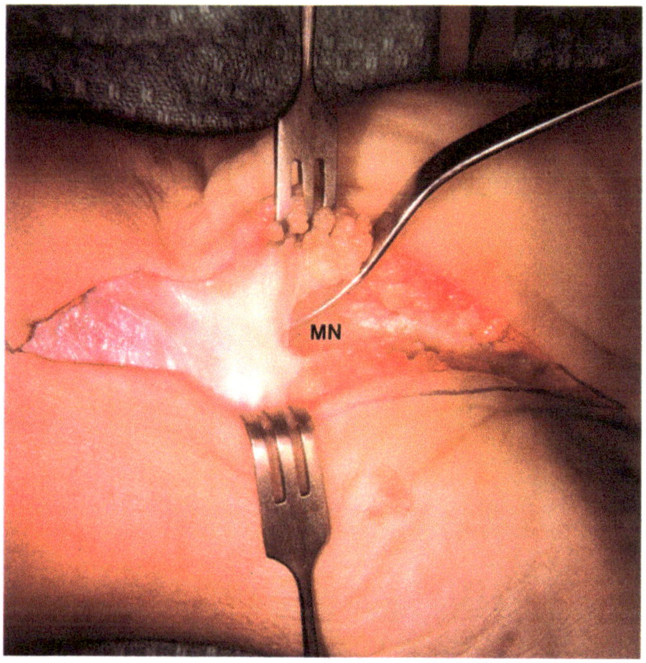

61 The deep fascia of the forearm forming the roof of a tunnel over the median nerve (MN) proximal to the flexor retinaculum.

Exposure of the median nerve

62 Exposure of the median nerve. Retract the wound edges to display the superficial contents of the carpal tunnel, the median nerve (1), and the nine flexor tendons (2). Note the superficial palmar arch distally (3).

Caution – Do not confuse the median nerve with the flexor tendon. The nerve can be distinguished by its colour (grey and dull compared to the white glistening tendon), consistency (softer), and the median artery (4) lying on its palmar surface.

Division of the flexor retinaculum and related fascia is not complete until the median nerve can be seen throughout its course in the canal.

Incomplete division of the flexor retinaculum is the commonest cause of failure of this operation.

The distal edge of the flexor retinaculum is the part most commonly left undivided.

Note the appearance of the median nerve (see page 17).

In this operation the median nerve is congested and slightly compressed by the flexor retinaculum. There is continuity of the median artery. There appears to be a significant amount of tenosynovium (5).

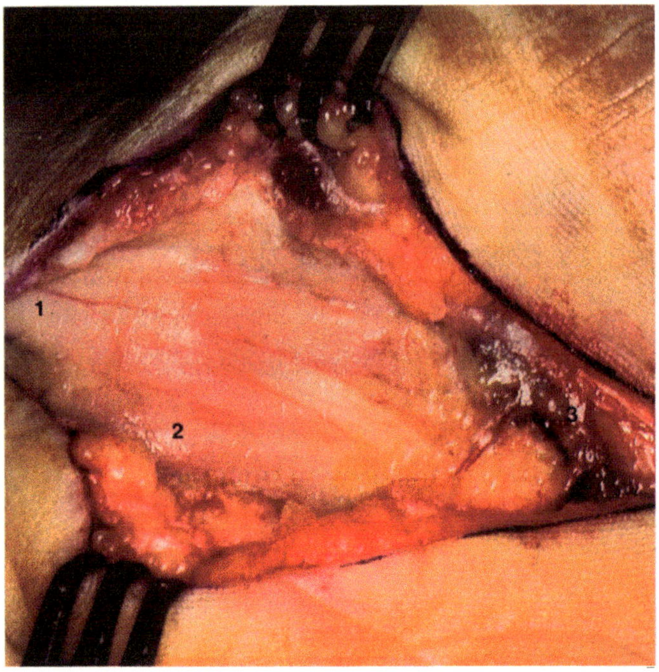

62

External median neurolysis

63
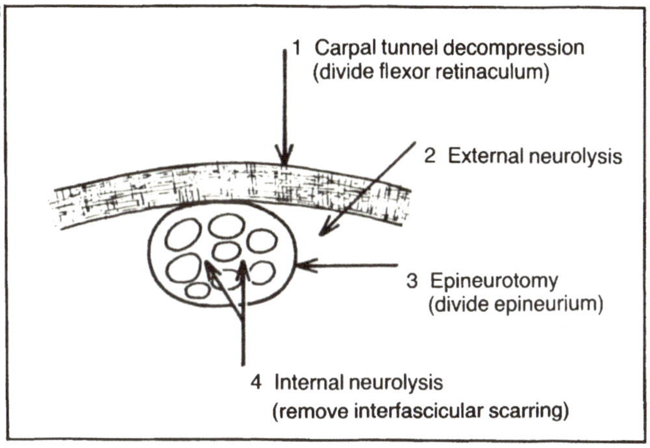

63 Types of operation for median nerve compression. 1 and 2 bring relief to most patients. 3 and 4 are potentially hazardous procedures and should only be performed by experienced surgeons. Of all the peripheral nerves the median nerve deserves the most consideration and the most delicate handling. Causalgia all too frequently results from minor trauma to the median nerve(84).

64a External median neurolysis. In some cases the median nerve is obscured and even compressed by a thick fascial layer deep to the flexor retinaculum.

64b Such a layer in this patient needed division before the condition of the median nerve could be accurately assessed. Note the median nerve here is congested and constricted.

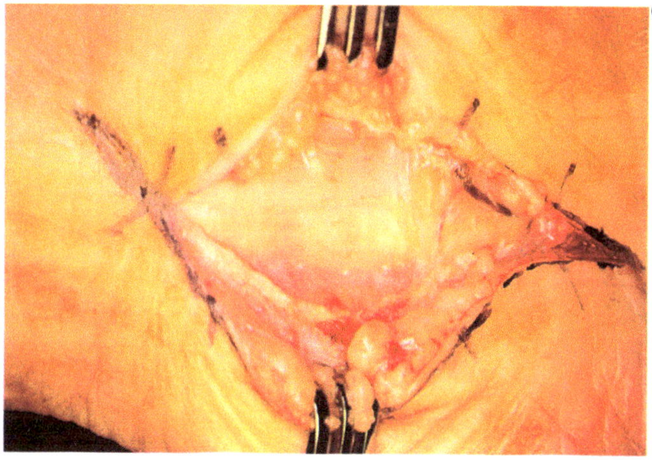
64a

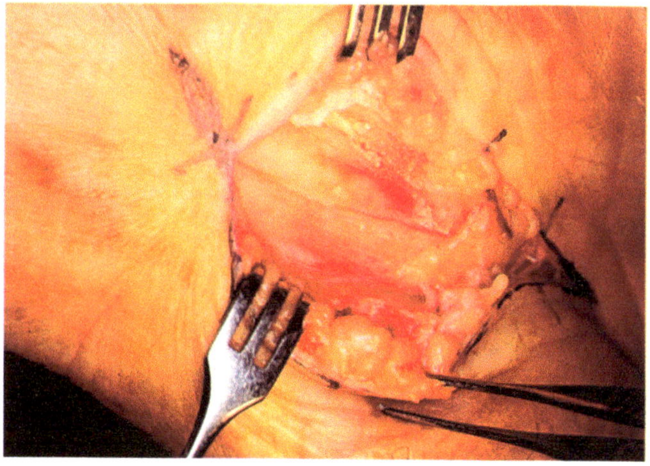
64b

65

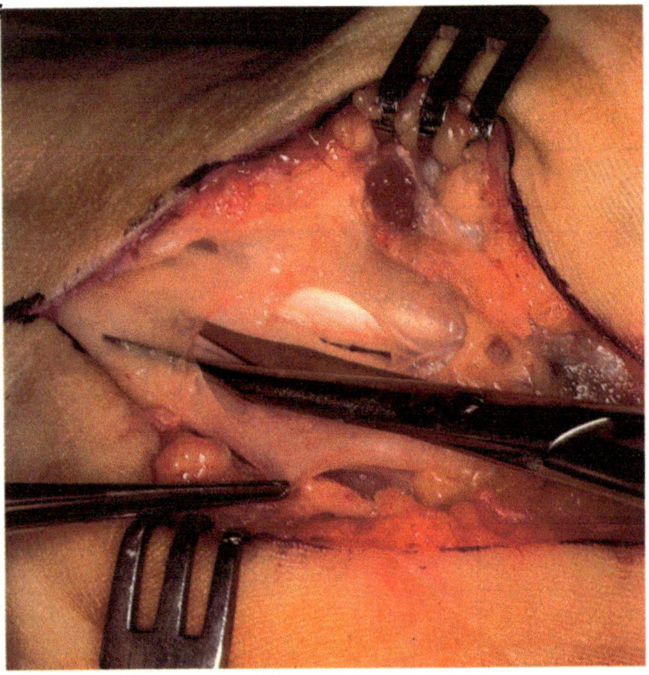

66

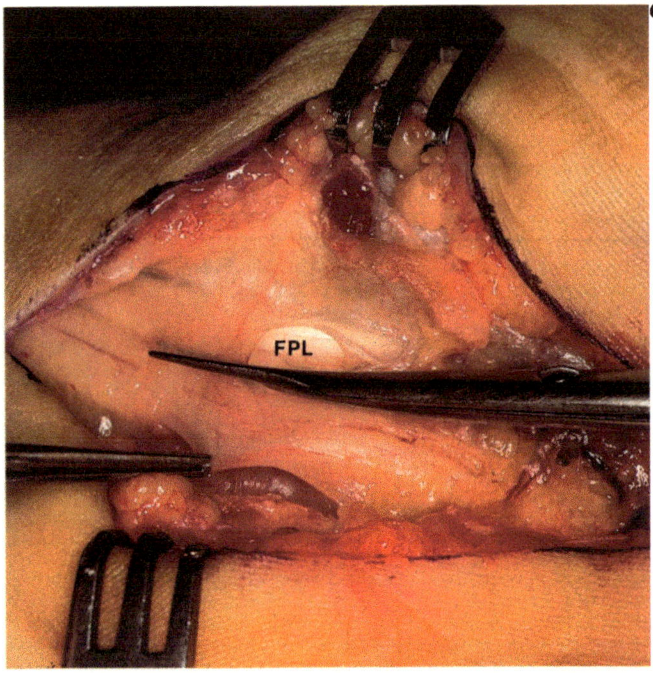

65 · External median neurolysis. Using fine dissecting forceps and scissors, dissect the fascial tissues superficial to the median nerve. Grasp the fascia around the nerve and not the nerve itself.

Note: Neurolysis is not a routine procedure. Division of the flexor retinaculum and the related fascia is usually sufficient.

Indications

1 If the median nerve is adherent to the deep surface of the flexor retinaculum or adjacent tendons.
2 If the median nerve is constricted by fascia.

66 Cut these tissues to free the median nerve from the surrounding tissues. The tendon of flexor pollicis longus (FPL) is seen on the radial side of the median nerve.

67

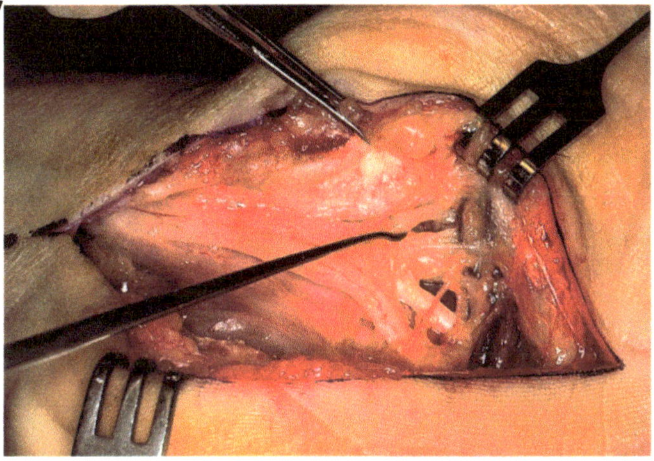

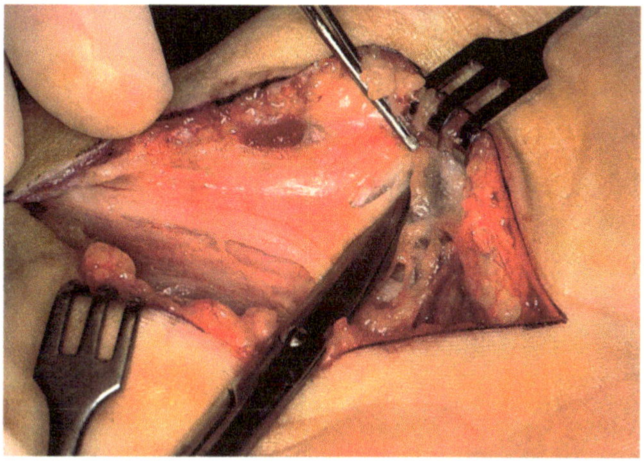

68a

67 Exposure of the terminal branches of the median nerve.

Indications Exposure and mobilisation of the terminal branches of the median nerve (MN) is not a necessary routine unless there has been selective impairment of a sensory digital branch or branches, or the recurrent thenar branch.

Technique Dissect from proximal to distal the trunk of the nerve as it divides into its five digital sensory branches and recurrent thenar motor branch. (Recurrent motor branch demonstrated by the hook retractor.)

Dissect in a longitudinal direction to avoid damage to the nerves and their blood supply.

68a Recurrent thenar branch. If there has been thenar muscle wasting and weakness or tenderness, retract the divided flexor retinaculum and gently dissect the recurrent thenar branch or branches into the thenar muscles.

Isolated involvement of this branch may occur as it angles over the distal margin of the flexor retinaculum or when it has an anomalous course through the ligament.

Release any compression of the branch by cutting the fascia superficial to it.

Caution – Beware of variations in the size, point of origin, and the course of the recurrent thenar motor branch (see **34**). *Neurolysis of this nerve is NOT a necessary routine.*

68b

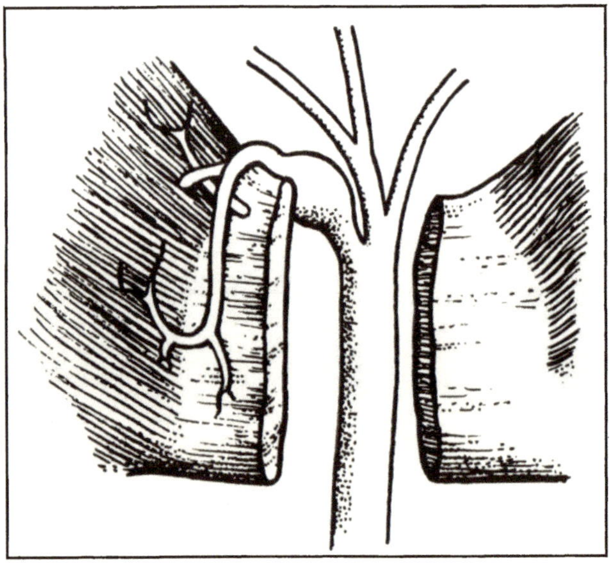

68b Recurrent motor branch compressed as it angles back over the distal edge of the flexor retinaculum.

Rationale(21) – Intraneural fibrosis may maintain compression of the axons after the flexor retinaculum has been divided.

Caution – This procedure is potentially hazardous. Postoperative interfascicular scarring can produce irreparable damage to the median nerve. More harm than good results unless the surgeon is experienced in microneural techniques.

Internal median neurolysis (endoneurolysis)

Indications

1 Motor and/or sensory loss caused by interruption of nerve conduction, for example, palsy of abductor pollicis brevis.
2 Persistent pain and paraesthesiae.
3 Operative findings of:
 – hour-glass constriction of the median nerve.
 – gross thickening of the epineurium.
 – palpable induration.
 – obliteration of the median artery.
4 Recurrent carpal tunnel syndrome.

69

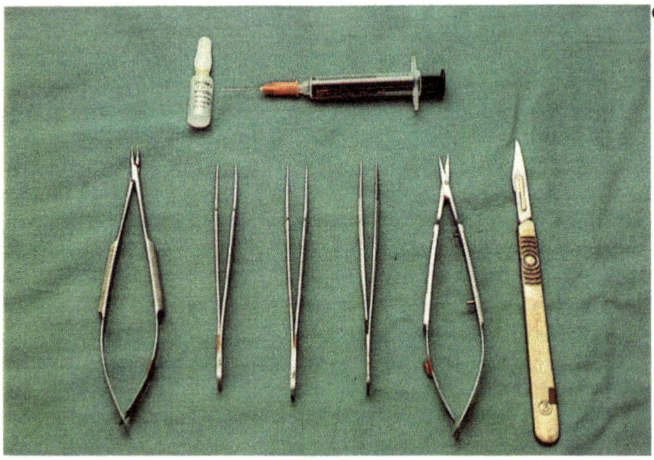

69 Instruments for internal neurolysis. (NB: magnification and fine microneural instruments are essential to the safe conduct of this meticulous procedure.) (see **41**)

70

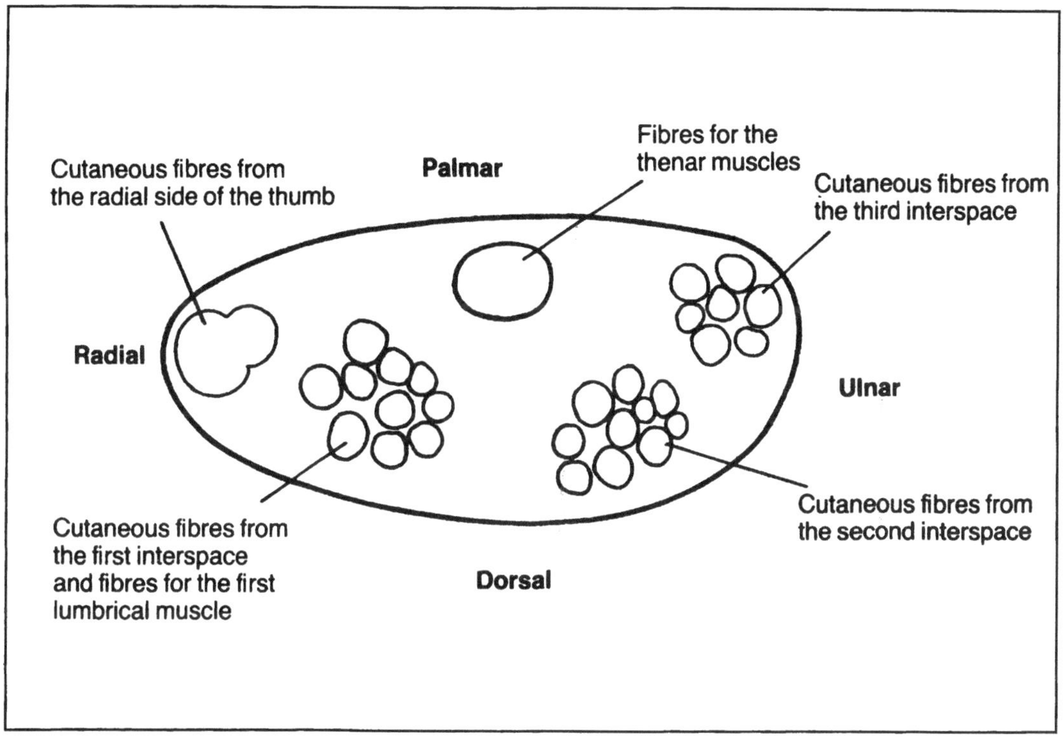

70 Orientation of fibres in the median nerve at the left wrist.

71a

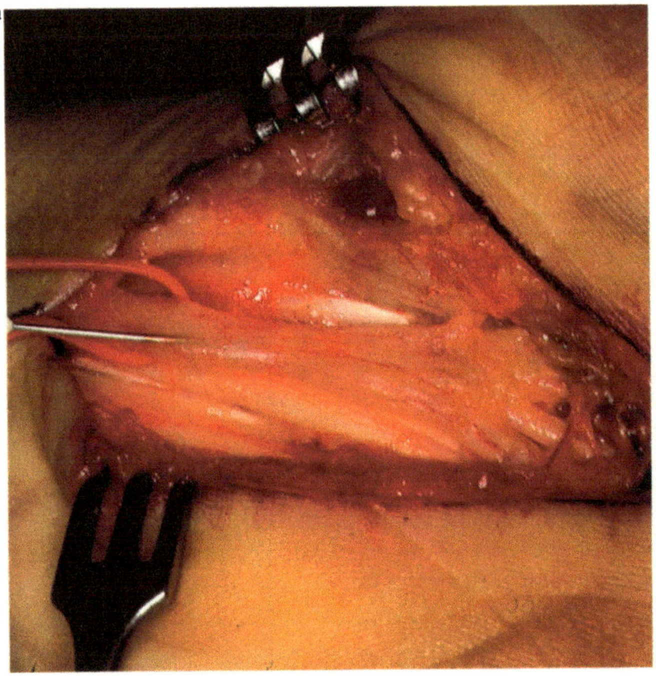

71b

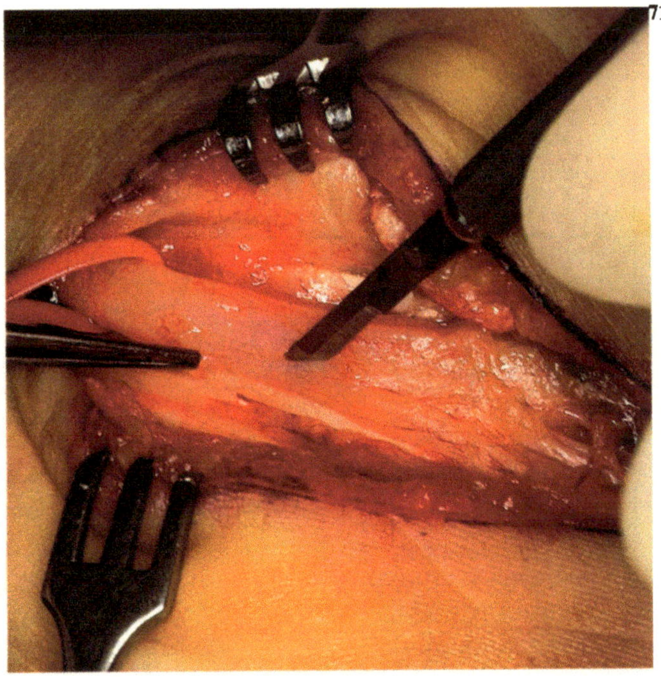

71a Use a 1 or 2 ml syringe and a very fine (25 to 30 gauge) hypodermic needle.

Inject a few drops of saline very slowly and gently deep to the epineural layer. This helps to separate the nerve bundles from the surrounding connective tissue.

The median nerve is supported by a soft rubber strip passed around it in the proximal part of the carpal tunnel.

Caution – Do not separate the nerve from its bed in the carpal tunnel. This might interfere with the circulation to the nerve. In traversing the carpal tunnel the median nerve lies in relatively avascular surroundings[8].

71b Tense the epineurium with micro-forceps. Use a fine scalpel blade or micro-scissors and incise the epineurium vertically across the constriction or indurated area.

Caution – Avoid damage to the neural vessels and so minimise the risk of intraneural haematoma or ischaemia. Minimal dissection will preserve the blood supply of the nerve.

Magnification and fine microneural instruments are essential to the safe conduct of this meticulous procedure.

72

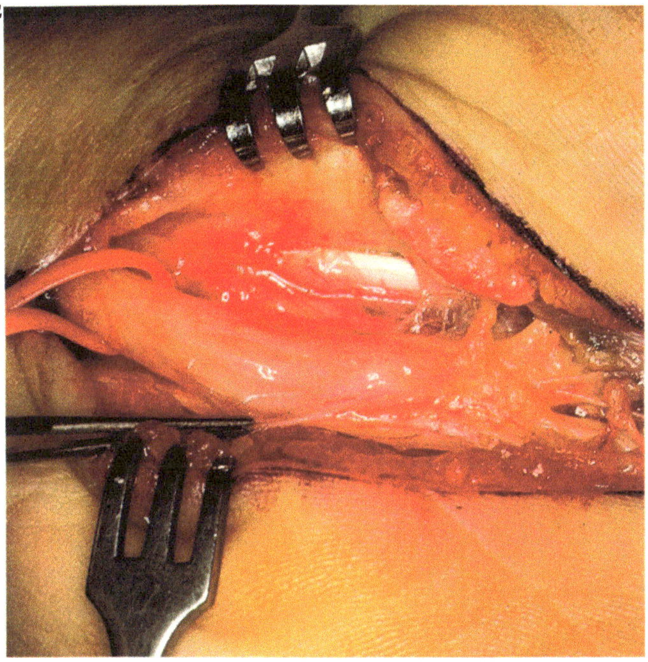

72 Use micro-forceps to retract the divided epineurium. Carry out sufficient dissection with magnification to delineate the fascicular groups of the median nerve (see **71**).

If interfascicular adhesions are abundant, then separate the fasciculi carefully with fine sharp instruments, under magnification, to avoid damage to them.

Limit the internal neurolysis to clinically involved funiculi, for example, in cases of thenar atrophy dissect the thenar fascicle. In cases when the middle finger is symptomatic, dissect the medial funiculi destined for the 2nd and 3rd web spaces.

Caution – This procedure demands experience in microneural techniques if irreversible iatrogenic damage to the median nerve is to be avoided. Do NOT perform internal neurolysis on all funiculi.

73

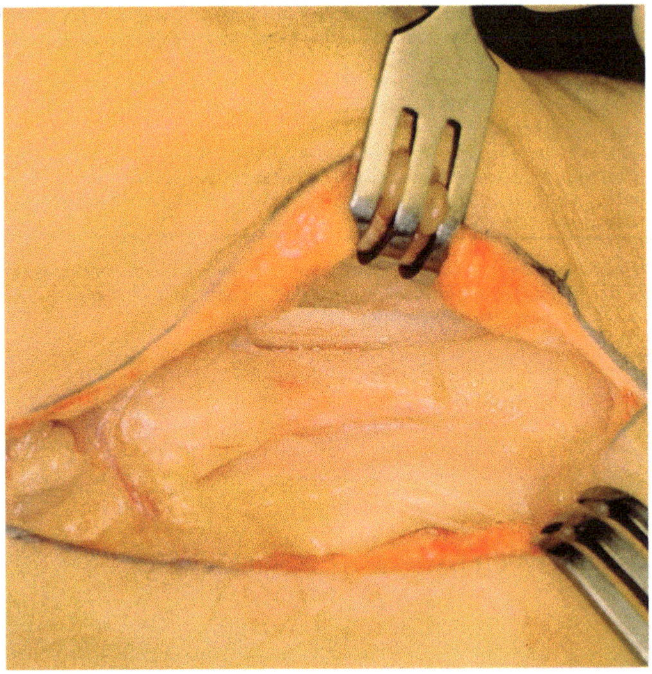

74

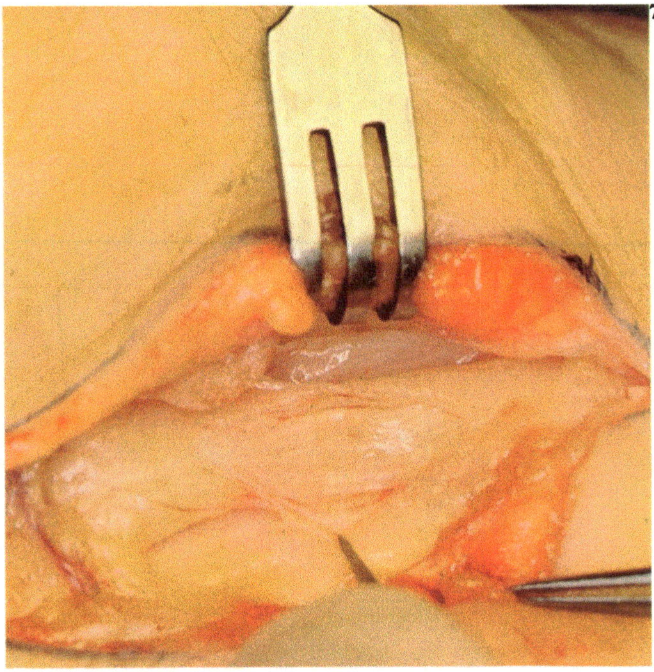

73 Constriction of the right median nerve in a patient with longstanding càrpal tunnel syndrome with thenar muscle weakness and wasting.

74 After epineurotomy and selective internal neurolysis.

Flexor tenosynovectomy

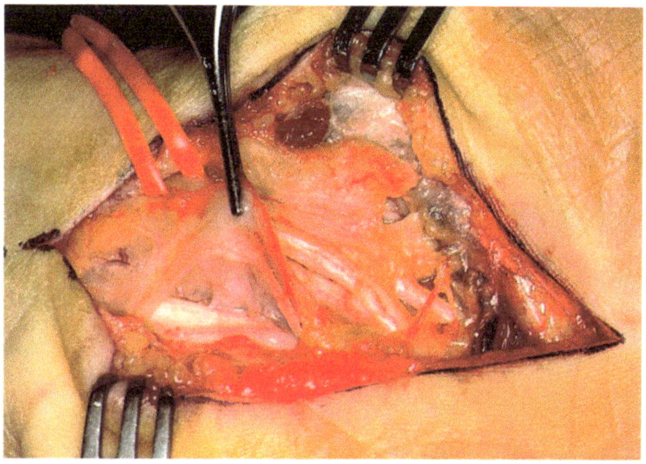
75

75 Flexor tenosynovectomy.
Indications Proliferative flexor tenosynovium which has persisted after adequate conservative measures and which:
(a) is grossly hypertrophied and compressing the median nerve;
(b) is interfering with the flexor tendon glide;
(c) is invading the substance of the flexor tendons.
Technique Protect and gently retract the median nerve with soft rubber tubing. Grasp the proliferative tenosynovium with dissecting forceps or haemostat.

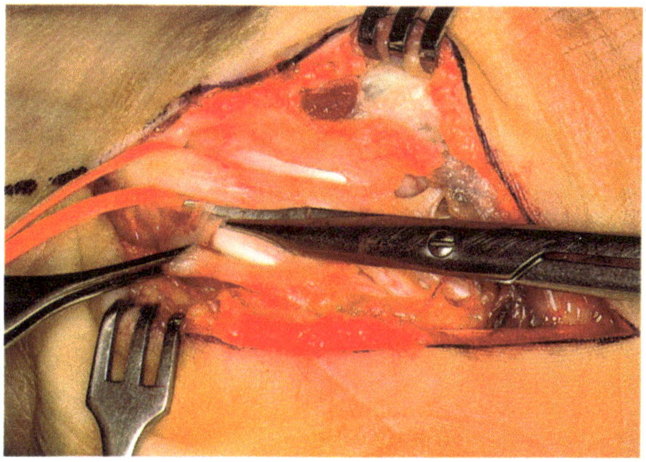
76

76 Cut along the flexor tendons and remove the involved flexor tenosynovium.
Extension of the wound into the distal forearm is usually required.

Caution – Excessive removal of synovium can create raw bleeding surfaces which heal by excessive scar, causing adhesions around the flexor tendons, with limitation of tendon glide and loss of grip strength.

Ulnar neurolysis

77 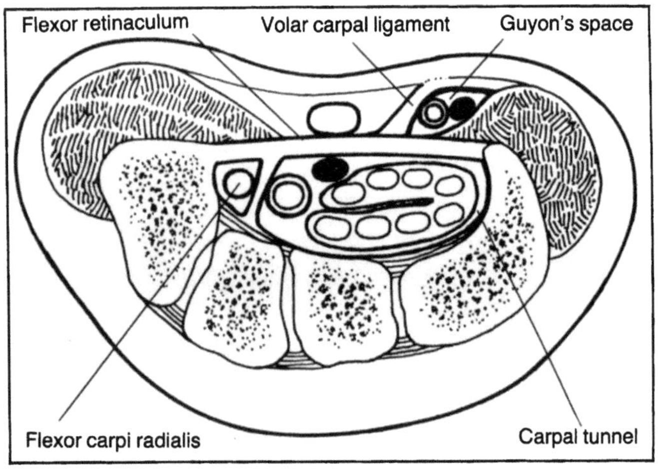

77 Cross section at the level of the wrist showing three tunnels. (1) The tunnel for flexor carpi radialis; (2) The carpal tunnel; (3) Guyon's space or loge (see also **3**).

Ulnar neurolysis in Guyon's space
Pathology A ganglion is the most common cause of compression of the ulnar nerve in this space(92). Proliferative flexor tenosynovium can also extend from the forearm into Guyon's space(104). Other causes include true or false aneurysms of the ulnar artery, thrombosis of the ulnar artery, fracture of the hook of the hamate with haemorrhage, lipoma or aberrant muscles pressing on the ulnar nerve.

Differential diagnosis. Exclude herniation of a cervical disc, thoracic outlet syndrome, peripheral neuritis, entrapment of the ulnar nerve at the elbow.

Indications for neurolysis. Clinical or EMG features of entrapment of the ulnar nerve at this level (see page 25).

Technique. Make the standard incision for carpal tunnel decompression (see **43, 44**). Guyon's space can be explored before or after opening the carpal tunnel.

78

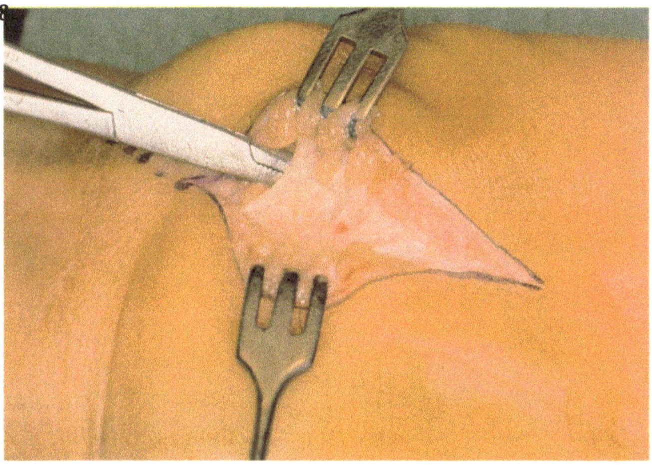

79

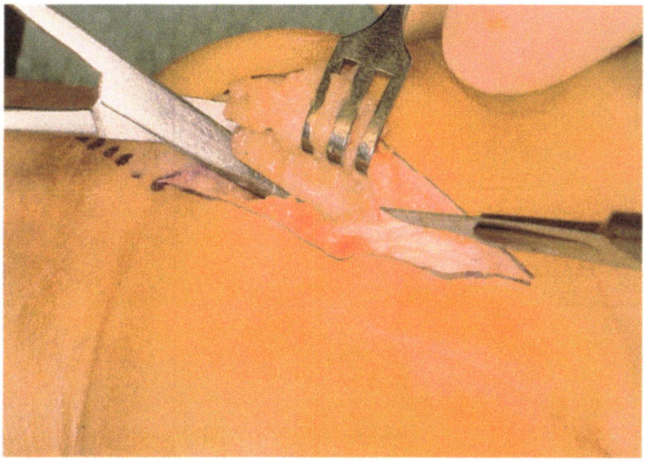

80

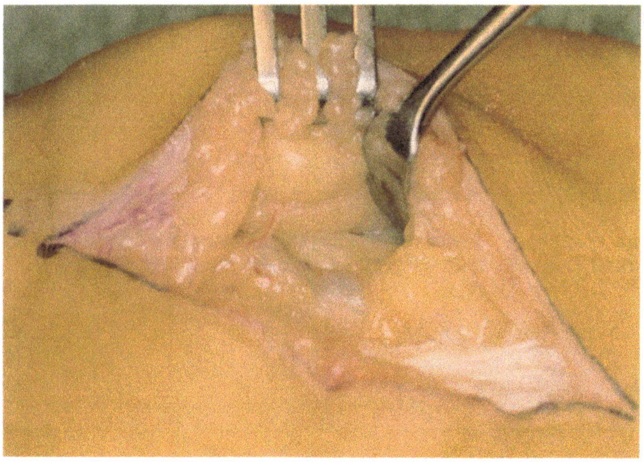

78 to 80 Ulnar neurolysis in Guyon's space before exploration of the carpal tunnel.

78 An artery forceps follows the course of the ulnar nerve in Guyon's space.

79 The space is opened by cutting the roof of the canal, i.e. the volar carpal ligament.

80 The ulnar neurovascular bundle. No compression was found.

81

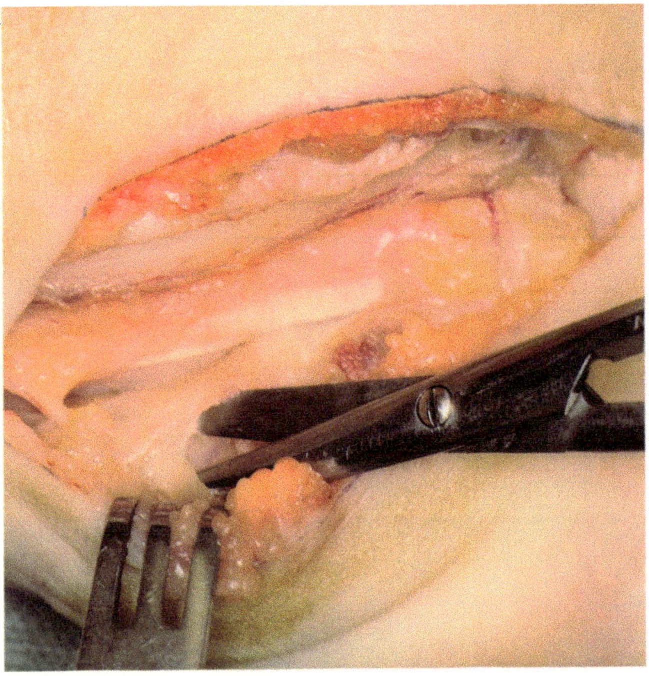

82

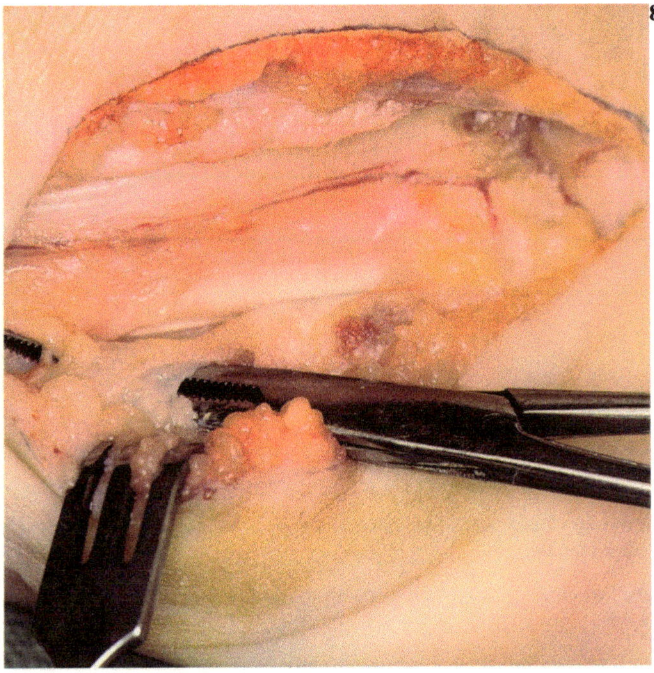

81 and 82 Ulnar neurolysis after exploration of the carpal tunnel.

81 Technique Retract the ulnar part of the wound and from either the distal or proximal part dissect the ulnar neurovascular bundle.

82 In this case there was free passage of an artery forceps superficial to the ulnar neurovascular bundle along Guyon's space.

Note the relatively thin volar carpal ligament which forms the roof of Guyon's space.

Operation for persistent or recurrent carpal tunnel syndrome

In **persistent carpal tunnel syndrome** the symptoms persist after carpal tunnel decompression. The most common cause is incomplete division of the flexor retinaculum.

In **recurrent carpal tunnel syndrome** the symptoms recur usually after about 3 months. The most common cause is fibrosis around the median nerve or hypertrophy of the flexor tenosynovium.

Indications for re-operation.
If the clinical features are compatible with the diagnosis of CTS, re-exploration of the carpal tunnel should be undertaken, regardless of the presence of a previous surgical scar[58].

Table 10.

Causes of unrelieved or recurrent carpal tunnel syndrome (CTS)
1 Incomplete division of flexor retinaculum
2 Hypertrophy of flexor teno synovium
3 Fibrous proliferation
(a) Within the carpal tunnel enmeshing median nerve or flexor tendons
(b) Reconstitution of flexor retinaculum itself

Table 11.

Surgical treatment of unrelieved or recurrent CTS
1 Divide flexor retinaculum
2 Neurolysis, external or internal
3 Tenosynovectomy
4 Instil corticosteroid into the wound

83

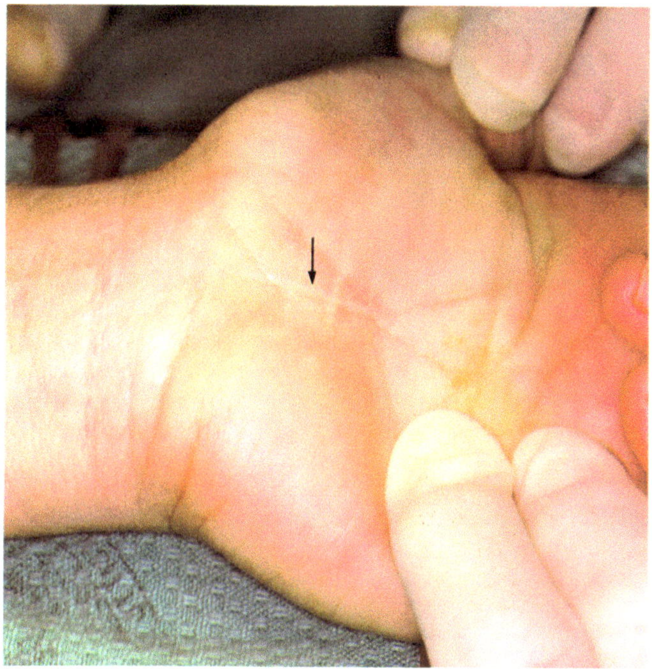

83 Recurrent carpal tunnel syndrome three months after carpal tunnel decompression through a short thenar incision (arrowed). Re-operation one year later.

Table 12.

Results of re-exploration[58]		
Good	Condition normal or 75 per cent improved	51 per cent
Fair	Improved 25–75 per cent	33 per cent
Poor	Unchanged or worsened	16 per cent

84

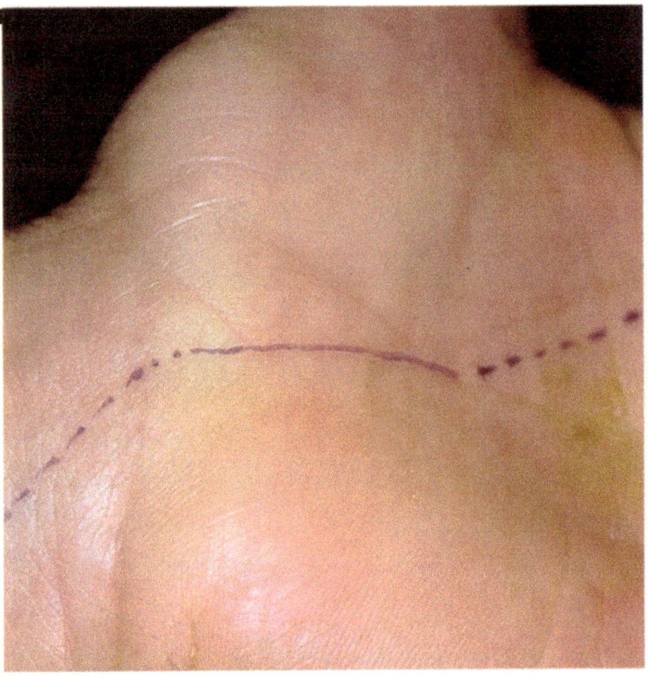

85

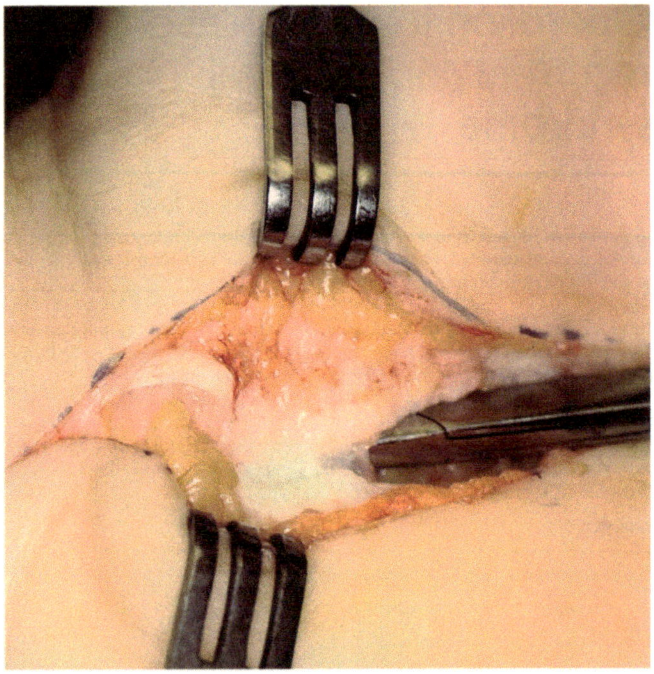

84 Line of incision to ensure complete division of the flexor retinaculum and its proximal and distal fascial attachments. Extend the wound as in this illustration, from the mid palm to 2 to 3 cm proximal to the wrist.

85 A haemostat in the carpal tunnel showing healing of the flexor retinaculum.

86

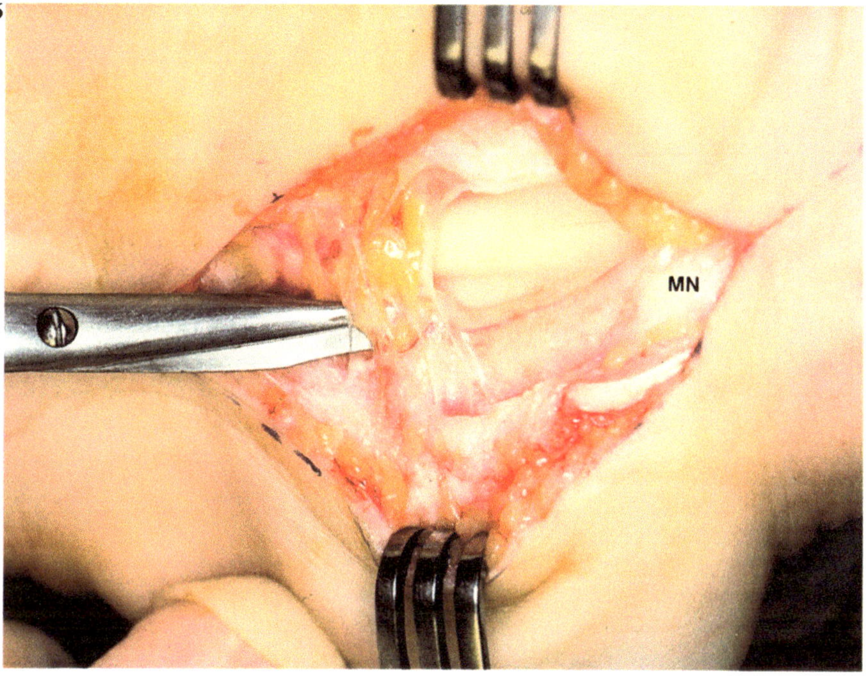

86 Cause of the recurrence: scarring and adhesions of the median nerve (MN).

Caution – Because of the distortion to the anatomy, be extra careful with the dissection. Find the median nerve in the normal unscarred tissues proximally and dissect distally.

87

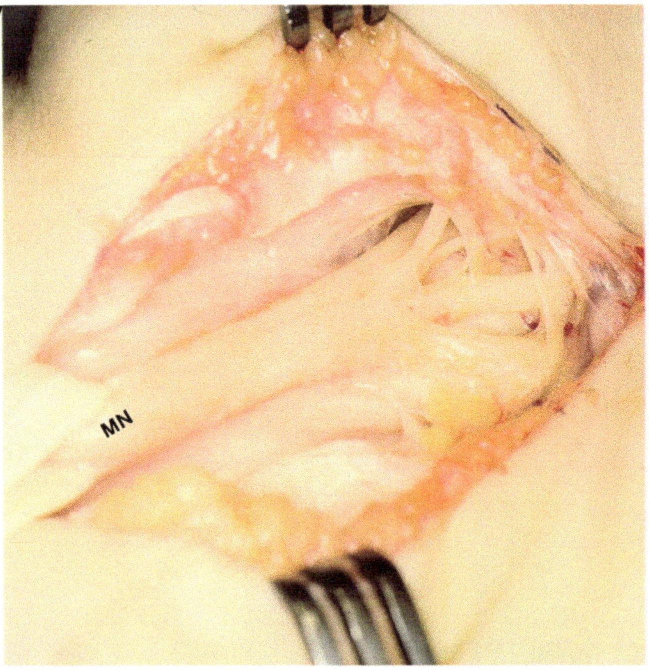

88

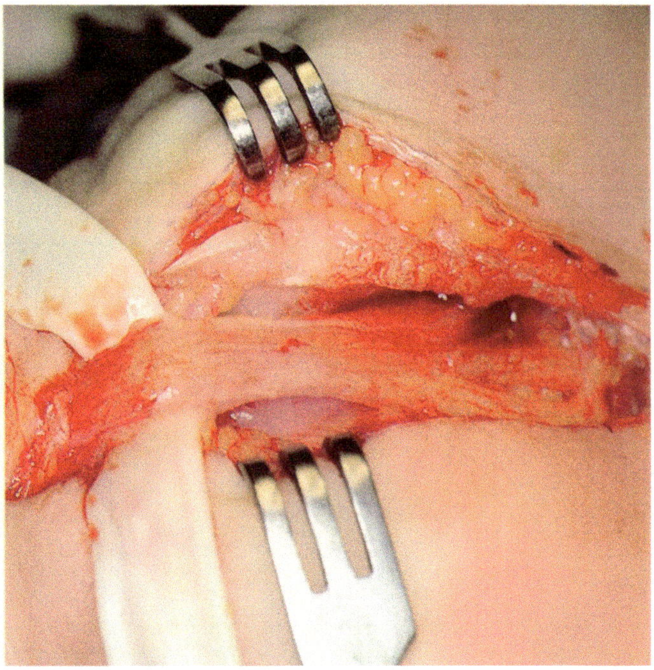

87 Dissect the median nerve (MN) and its branches as previously described under Median Neurolysis.

An internal median neurolysis was not performed in this case, because the median nerve felt soft; under magnification the fascicles could be seen throughout the length of the median nerve in the canal.

88 Release the tourniquet. Compress the wound. Elevate the hand. Wait five minutes. Ligate or coagulate any persistent bleeding points.

89

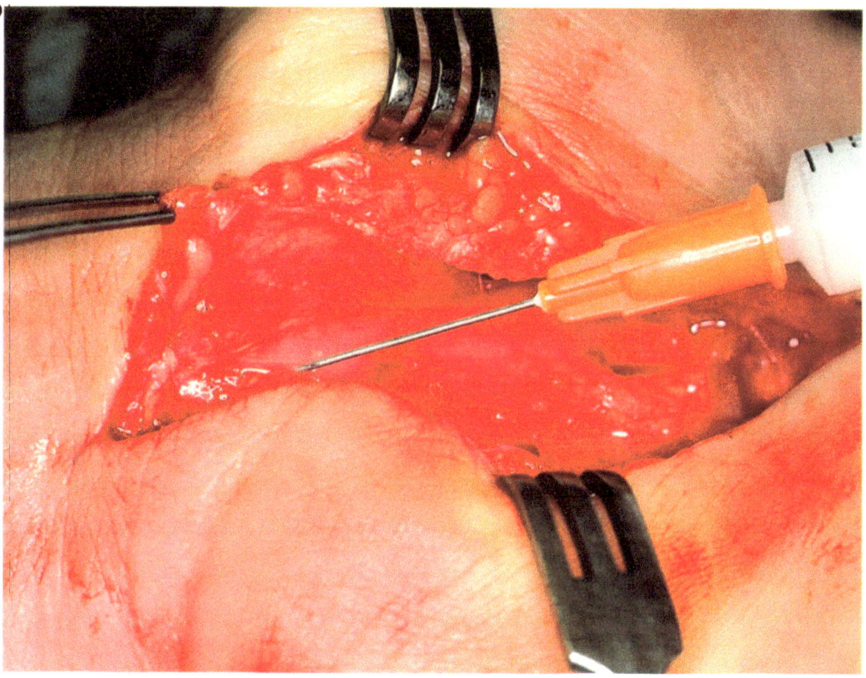

89 Perfuse corticosteroids (triamcinolone) into the wound before closure, to minimise scar formation around the separated fascicles.

90

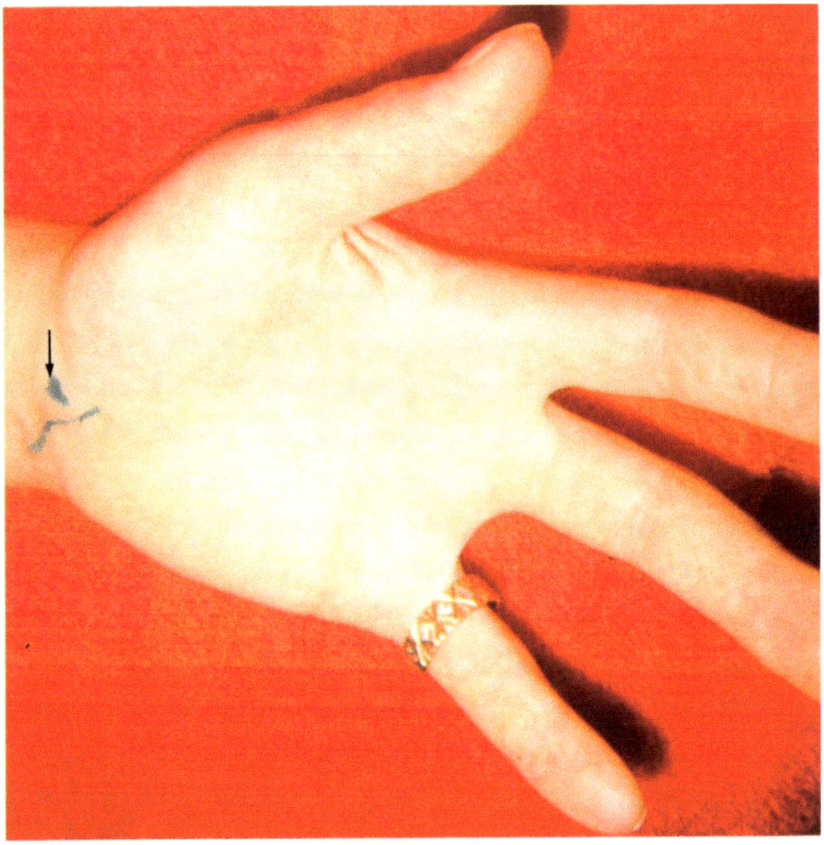

90 Persistent carpal tunnel syndrome. After failed replantation of her left ring finger, this 23-year-old nurse developed carpal tunnel syndrome and had surgical decompression. The short oblique incision gave direct exposure only to the proximal part of the carpal tunnel.
The arrow points to the pseudo-neuroma of the median nerve.

91

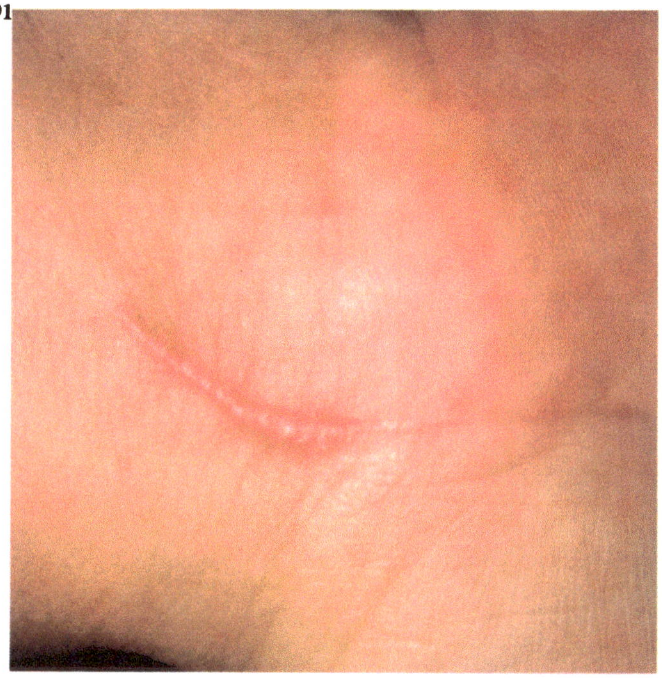

92

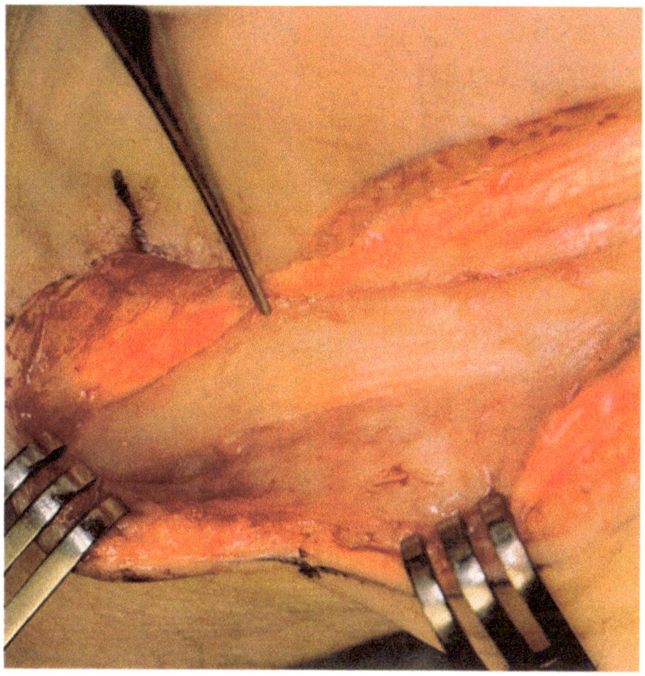

91 Persistent carpal tunnel syndrome. Three days after closed reduction and plaster immobilisation for a Colles' fracture, this 33-year-old surveyor had carpal tunnel decompression. The incision gave direct exposure only to the proximal part of the carpal tunnel.

92 Re-operation at nine months. The median nerve was severely compressed and fibrosed beneath the distal half of the flexor retinaculum. An internal neurolysis was required.

Reconstruction of the flexor retinaculum

The function of the flexor retinaculum is to maintain the transverse carpal arch and support the carpus. It also protects the median nerve and serves as a pulley for the flexor tendons. Although the divided flexor retinaculum will heal by scar, some surgeons advise reconstruction of the flexor retinaculum. This may be done by developing fascial flaps with a distal base on one side and a proximal base on the other. These are sutured side by side across the tunnel. The product is a new ligament approximately 2 cm wide with adequate clearance of the contents of the tunnel[50].

Tendon transfer for opposition of the thumb

When a carpal tunnel syndrome is associated with symptomatic thenar palsy of more than 12 months' duration (the patient being unable to oppose the thumb), consideration is given to opposition tendon transfer at the time of carpal tunnel decompression. With the carpal tunnel open and the flexor retinaculum divided, the palmaris longus can be taken with a distal strip of palmar aponeurosis attached to it, and transferred to the tendon of insertion of abductor pollicis brevis[10]. Alternatively the flexor superficialis of the ring finger can be taken as a donor unit[43].

Exploration of the carpal tunnel floor

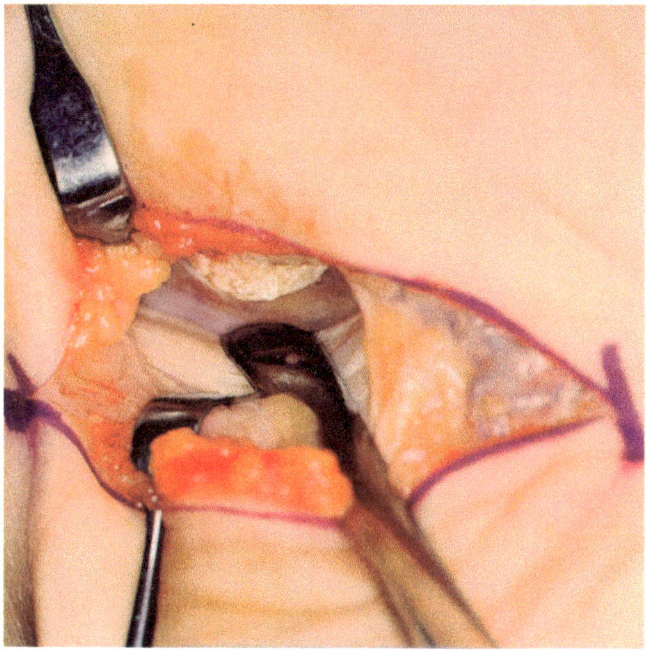

93b

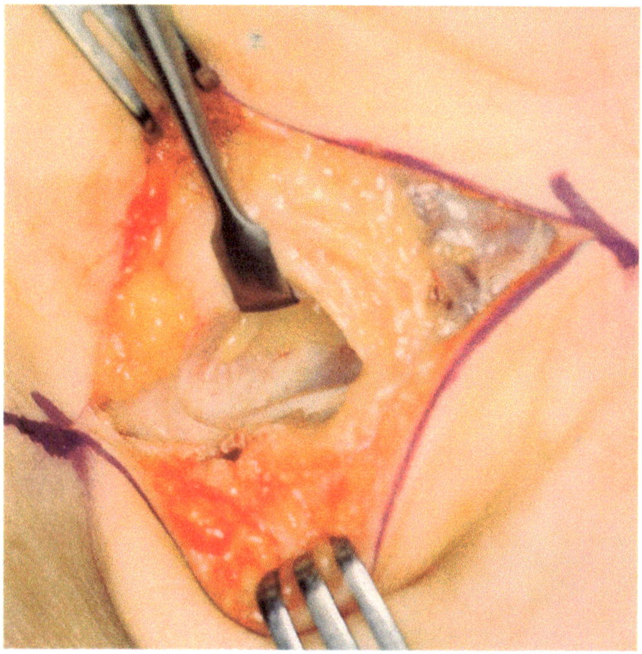

93a and b Exploration of the carpal tunnel floor. Protect the median nerve and retract the flexor tendons, first to the radial and then to the ulnar side, to examine the volar aspect of the wrist joint, i.e. the floor of the carpal tunnel. Look for:

1 A space-occupying lesion, for example, ganglion or lipoma, abnormal muscle.

2 Bony spicules which might predispose to tendon rupture[75].

EXPLORATION OF THE CARPAL TUNNEL FLOOR

94 Ganglion arising from the intercarpal joints and pressing on the radial division of the median nerve in the carpal tunnel.

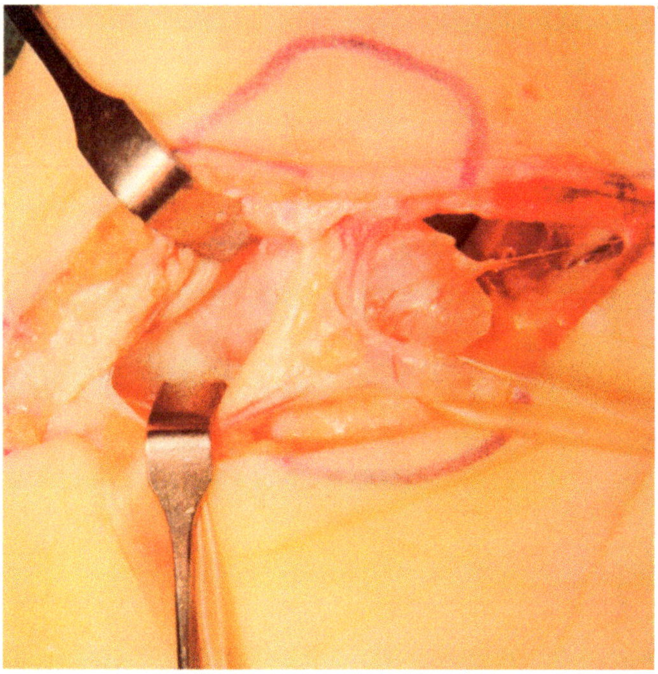
94

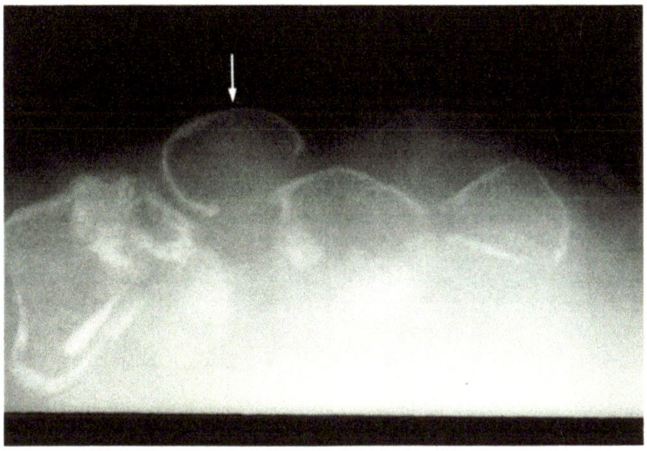

95 A carpal tunnel view. This rheumatoid arthritis patient suffered from carpal tunnel syndrome. Sharp bony spicules arising from the carpal tunnel floor gave rise to rupture of the flexor pollicis longus and flexor profundus of the index and middle fingers.

The arrow points to the sheeting of Silastic wrapped round the repaired tendons.

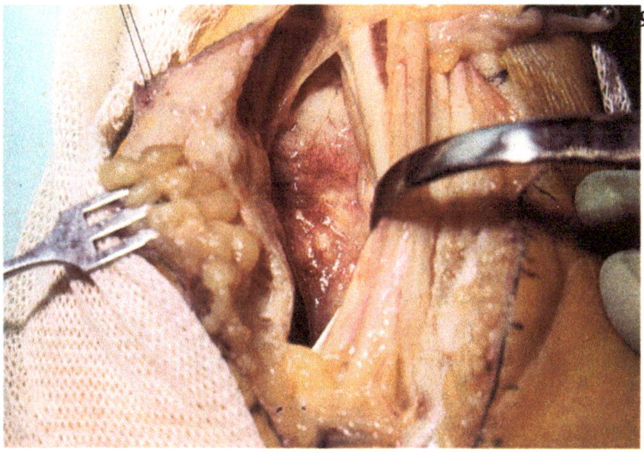

96

96 Gout. Urate crystals on the palmar aspect of the capsule of the wrist joint.

Wound closure

97

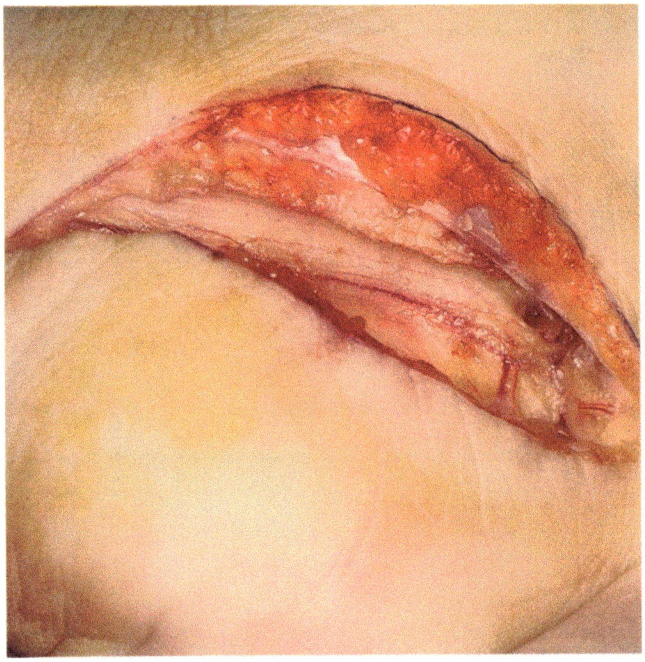

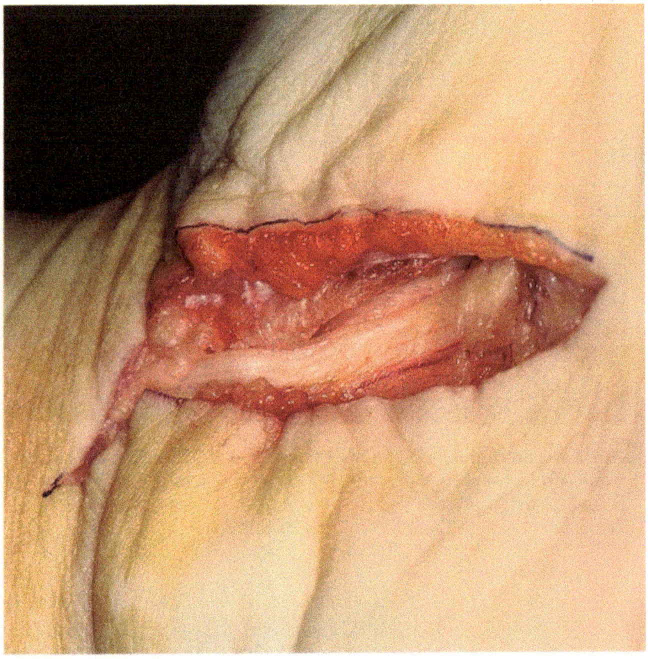

97 Preparation for wound closure. Position the wrist so that it is in neutral or slight extension and in slight ulnar deviation, so that the median nerve lies in the carpal tunnel and beneath the radial portion of the divided flexor retinaculum.

Palmaris longus If the palmaris longus tendon appears to compress the median nerve, sever the tendon at its insertion and resect a portion of it.

Tourniquet The tourniquet need only be released before wound closure if there is a risk of bleeding; e.g. after tenosynovectomy or re-operation with internal neurolysis.

98 Warning. If this patient's wound had been sutured and splinted in this position, the median nerve would have become adherent to the wound.

This is a cause of recurrence of median nerve symptoms.

99

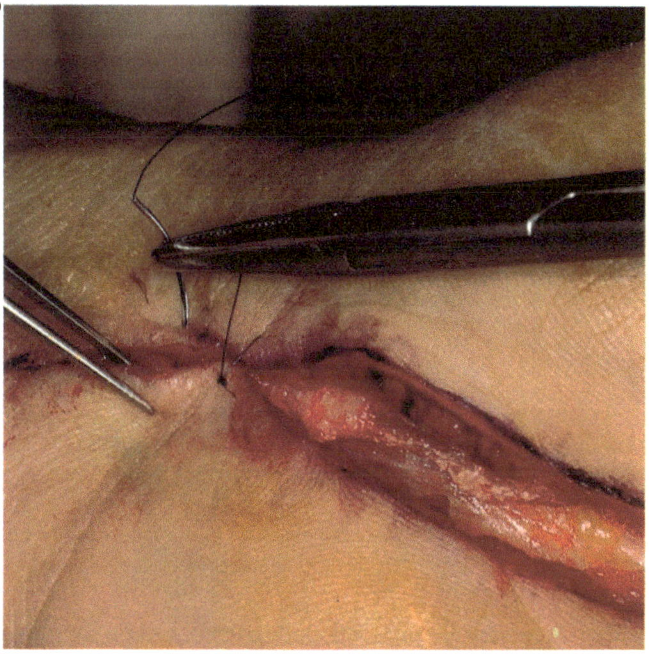

99 Wound closure. Close only the skin. Use atraumatic interrupted 5/0 nylon or other monofilament sutures. Begin by aligning the wrist crease.

100

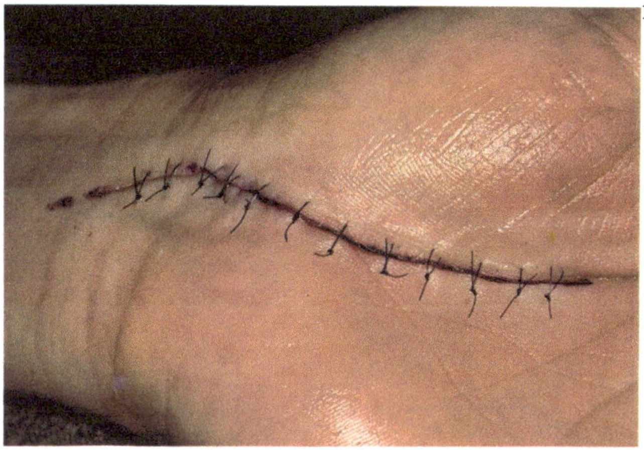

100 The sutured wound.

Dressing technique

101

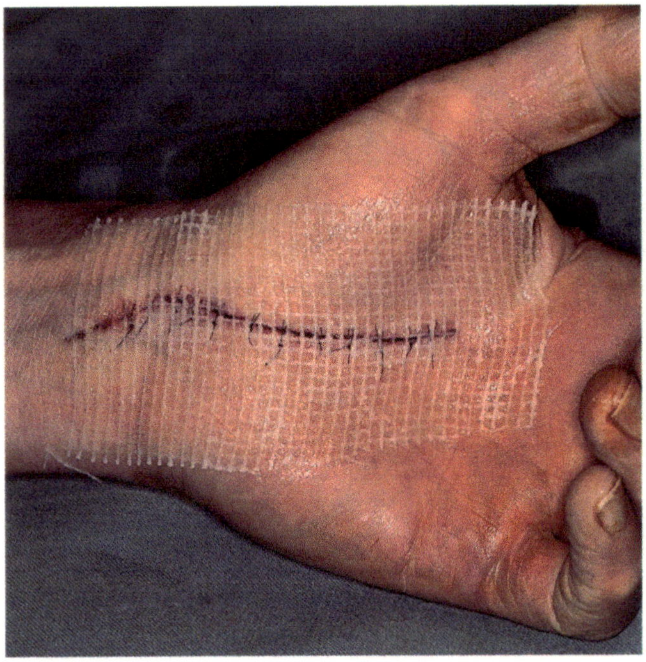

101 Dressing technique. Cover the wound with a single layer of vaseline gauze. Apply cotton gauze for compression and absorption.

102

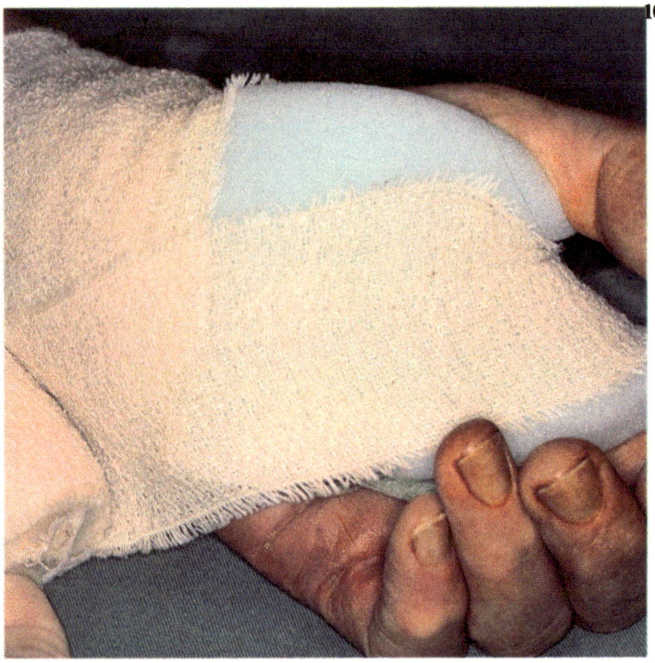

102 Cover with 1 cm thick polyurethane foam to protect the wound and the borders of the hand. Apply a 5 cm crêpe bandage.

Splintage

103
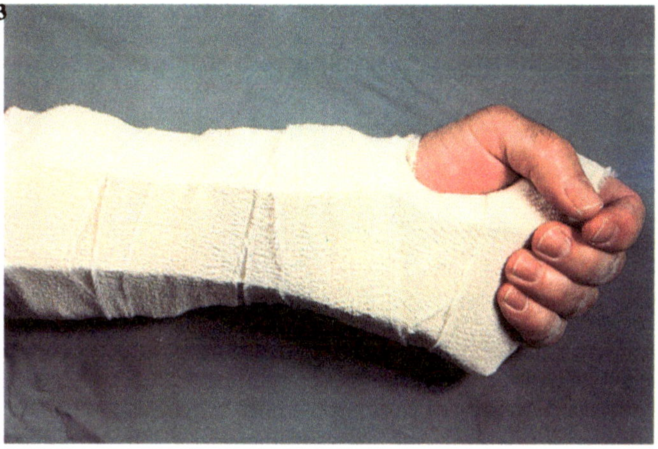

104
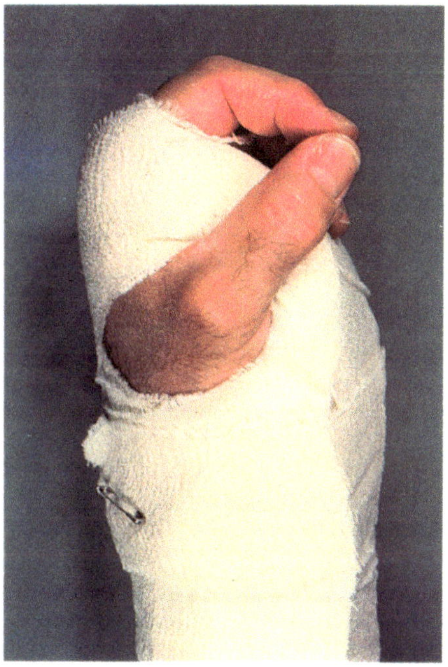

103 Plaster splint. Next make a 15 cm plaster of Paris slab to extend from two to three fingers distal to the elbow, and carry this plaster slab to the distal palmar crease, supporting the wrist in slight extension and ulnar deviation. Leave the fingers free to move at the interphalangeal joints.

104 Reinforce the plaster for extra strength.
The fingers should be free to move at the interphalangeal joints. The elbow must also be free.
Avoid plaster pressure on the thenar eminence.

105 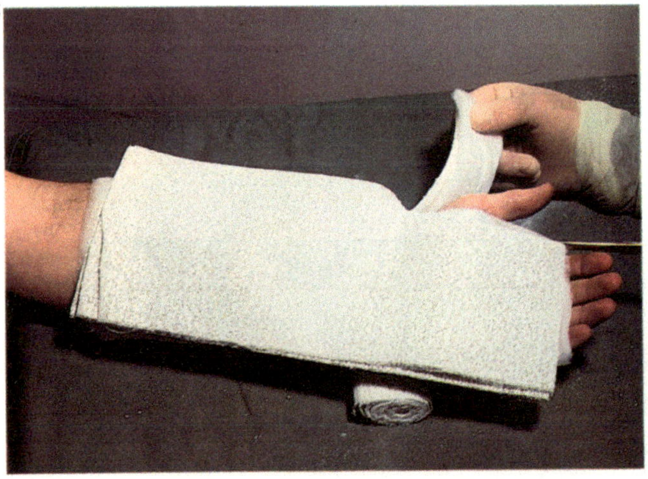

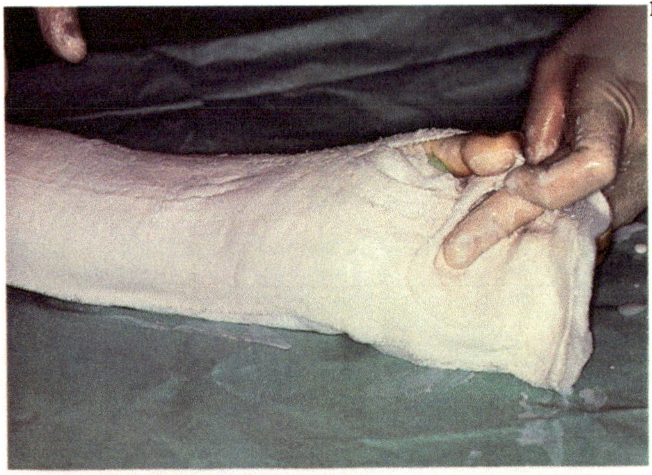 106

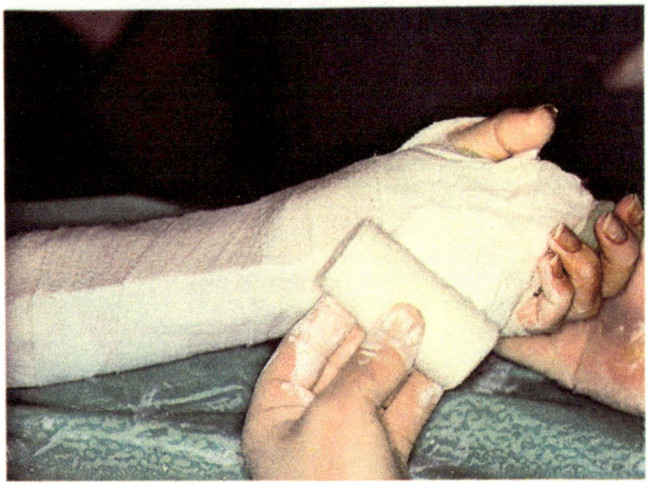 107

105 An alternate plaster immobilising technique. Measure a plaster slab from well below the elbow to just beyond the fingertips. The elbow should be flexed while the plaster is soft. Cut a longitudinal strip for the thumb about 3 cm wide, extending to the base of the thumb metacarpal.

106 Fold this strip across the extensor aspect of the metacarpophalangeal joint of the thumb to the mid-palm. This prevents full thumb extension and abduction but allows flexion and opposition.

107 Fold the finger section of the plaster back over the thumb strip at the level of the metacarpophalangeal joints. The fingers are free to move at the interphalangeal joints.

Postoperative care

108

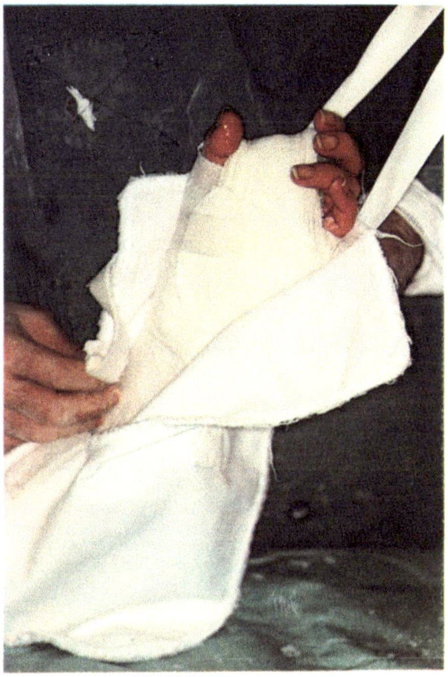

109

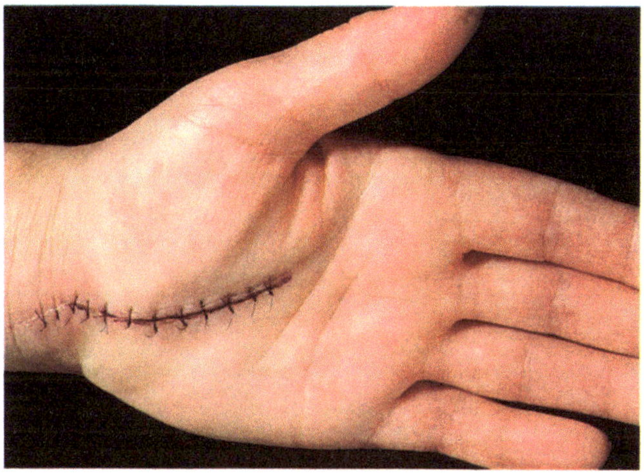

110

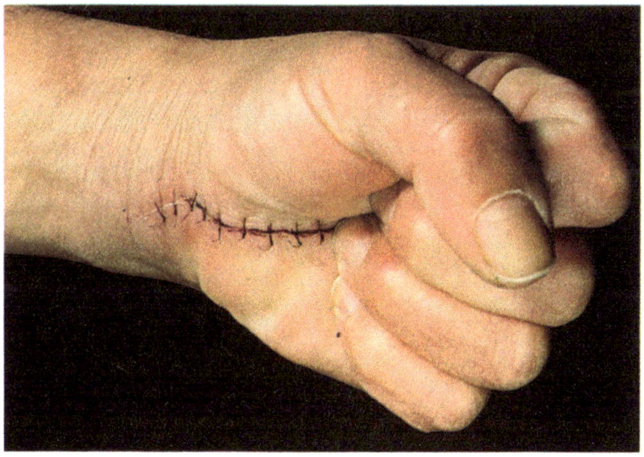

108 Before removing the tourniquet, support the forearm and hand in a sling and maintain this elevation for two or three days.

After release of the tourniquet, always check the circulation to the fingers.

109 At two weeks remove the dressing. Figures **109** and **110** show the degree of finger and thumb movement that should be attainable at this time.

110 Full flexion.

Remove the sutures and apply a firm bandage for support for another two weeks.

References

1 Abbott, Le Roy C. & Saunders, J.B. De C.M. (1933). 'Injuries of the median nerve in fractures of the lower end of the radius', *Surg Gynecol Obstet*, **57**, 507.

2 Adams, R., Jones, G. & Marble, H.C. (1940). 'Tuberculous tenosynovitis', *N Engl J Med*, **223**, 706.

3 Adamson, J.E., Srougi, S.J., Horton, C.E. & Maldick, R.A. (1971). 'The acute carpal tunnel syndrome', *Plast Reconstr Surg*, **47**, 332.

4 Artlet, J., Ficat, P. & Martinex, J. (1958). 'Carpal tunnel syndrome caused by compression during a severe tophaceous gout', *Revue rheum*, **25**, 581.

5 Ashby, B.S. (1964). 'Hypertrophy of the palmaris longus muscle' (Report of a case), *J Bone Joint Surg*, **46-B**, 230.

6 Backhouse, K.M. & Davidson, D.C. (1975). 'Anomalous palmaris longus muscle producing carpal tunnel like compression', *Hand*, **7**, 22.

7 Barber, K.W. Jun., Bianco, A.J., Soule, E.H. & Macarty, C.S. (1962). 'Benign extraneural soft tissue tumours of the extremities causing compression of nerves', *J Bone Joint Surg*, **44-A**, 98.

8 Blunt, M.J. (1959). 'The vascular anatomy of the median nerve in the forearm and hand', *J Anat*, **93**, 15.

9 Brain, W.R., Wright, A.D. & Wilkinson, M. (1947). 'Spontaneous compression of both median nerves in the carpal tunnel' (Six cases treated surgically), *Lancet*, **1**, 277.

10 Braun, R.M. (1978). 'Palmaris longus tendon transfer for augmentation of the thenar musculature in low median palsy', *J Hand Surg*, **3**, 488.

11 Brooks, D.M. (1952). 'Nerve compression by simple ganglia', *J Bone Joint Surg*, **34-B**, 391.

12 Burnham, P.J. (1963). 'Acute carpal tunnel syndrome: median artery thrombosis as cause', *Arch Surg*, **87**, 645.

13 Campbell, E.D.R. (1962). 'The carpal tunnel syndrome: investigation and assessment of treatment', *Proc Roy Soc Med*, **55**, 401.

14 Cannon, B.W. & Love, J.C. (1946). 'Tardy median palsy, median neuritis, median thenar neuritis amenable to surgery', *Surgery*, **20**, 210.

15 Carroll, R.E. & Green, D.P. (1972). 'The significance of the palmar cutaneous nerve at the wrist', *Clin Orthop*, **83**, 24.

16 Chalmers, T.M. cha. 26. In: Lamb, D.W. & Kuczynski, K. *The Principles of Hand Surgery*, Blackwell, Oxford, 1981.

17 Cherington, M. (1974). 'Proximal pain in carpal tunnel syndrome', *Arch Surg*, **108**, 69.

18 Conolly, W.B. (1978). 'Pitfalls in carpal tunnel decompression', *Aust NZ J Surg*, **48**, 421.

19 Crow, R.S. (1980). 'Treatment of carpal tunnel syndrome', *Brit Med J*, **1**, 1611.

20 Cseuz, K.A., Thomas, J.E., Lambert, E.H., Love, J.G. & Lipscomb, P.R. (1966). 'Long term results of operation for carpal tunnel syndrome', *Mayo Clin Proc*, **41**, 232.

21 Curtis, R.C. & Eversman, W.W. (1973). 'Internal neurolysis as an adjunct to the treatment of the carpal tunnel syndrome', *J Bone Joint Surg*, **55-A**, 737.

22 Das, S.K. & Brown, H.G. (1976). 'In search of complications in carpal tunnel decompression', *Hand*, **8**, 243.

23 Dekel, S., Papaioannou, T., Rushworth, G. & Coates, R. (1980). 'Idiopathic carpal tunnel stenosis', *Brit Med J*, **280**, 1297.

24 Earl, C.J., Gullerton, P.M., Wakefield, G.S. & Schutta, H.S. (1964). 'Hereditary neuropathy with liability to pressure palsies', *Q J Med*, **33**, 481.

25 Entin, M.A. (1968). 'Carpal tunnel syndrome and its variants', *Surg Clin North Am*, **48**, 1097.

26 Frank, D.H. (1981). 'Carpal and Guyon tunnel syndrome', *J Hand Surg*, **6**, 412.

27 Fullerton, P.M. (1963). 'The effect of ischaemia on nerve conduction in the carpal tunnel syndrome', *J Neurol Neurosurg Psychiatry*, **26**, 385.

28 Gainer, J.V. Jun., Nugent, G.R. (1977). 'Carpal tunnel syndrome: report of 430 operations', *South Med J*, **70**, 325.

29 Garland, H., Bradshaw, J.P. & Clark, J.M. (1957). 'Compression of the median nerve in the carpal tunnel and its relation to acroparaesthesiae', *Brit Med J*, **1**, 730.

30 Gelberman, R.H., Aronson, D. & Weisman, M.H. (1980). 'Carpal tunnel syndrome. Results of a prospective trial of steroid injection and splinting', *J Bone Joint Surg*, **62-A**, 1181.

31 Gelberman, R.H., Hergenroeder, P.T., Hargens, A.R., Lundborg, G.N. & Akeson, W.H. (1981). 'The carpal tunnel syndrome: a study of carpal canal pressures', *J Bone Joint Surg*, **63-A**, 380.

32 Gilliatt, R.W. & Sears, T.A. (1958). 'Sensory nerve action potentials in patients with peripheral nerve lesions', *J Neurol Neurosurg Psychiatry*, **21**, 109.

33 Gilliatt, R.W. & Willison, R.G. (1962). 'Peripheral nerve conduction in diabetic neuropathy', *J Neurol Neurosurg Psychiatry*, **25**, 11.

34 Gilliatt, R.W. & Wilson, T.G. (1953). 'A pneumatic tourniquet test in the carpal tunnel syndrome', *Lancet*, **2**, 595.

35 Goodman, H.V. & Gilliatt, R.W. (1961). 'The effect of treatment on median nerve conduction in patients with carpal tunnel syndrome', *Ann Phys Med*, **6m**, 137.

36 Goodwill, C.J. (1965). 'The carpal tunnel syndrome. Long term follow up showing of latency measurement to response to treatment', *Ann Phys Med*, **8**, 12.

37 Guyon, F. (1961). 'Note sure une disposition anatomique propre a las face anterieure de la region due poignet et non encore decrite', *Bull Soc Anatomique*, **36**, 184.

38 Heathfield, K.W.G. (1957). 'Acroparaesthesiae and the carpal tunnel syndrome', *Lancet*, **2**, 663.

39 Herndon, J.H., Eaton, R.G. & Litter, J.W. (1974). 'Carpal tunnel syndrome. An unusual presentation of osteoid osteoma', *J Bone Joint Surg*, **56-A**, 1715.

40 Hongell, A. & Mattsson, H.S. (1971). 'Neurographic studies before, after, and during operation for median nerve compression in the carpal tunnel', *Scand J Plast Resonstr Surg*, **5**, 103.

41 Hunt, J.R. (1911). 'The thenar and hypothenar types of neural atrophy of the hand', *Am J Med Sci*, **141**, 224.

42 Hybbinette, C.H. & Mannerfelt, L. (1975). 'The carpal tunnel syndrome – a retrospective study of 400 operated patients', *Acta Orthop Scand*, **46**, 610.

43 Inglis, A.E., Straub, L.R. & Williams, C.S. (1972). 'Median nerve neuropathy at the wrist', *Clin Orthop*, **83**, 48.

44 Jabaley, M.E. (1978). 'Personal observations on the role of the lumbrical muscles in carpal tunnel syndrome', *J Hand Surg*, **3**, 82.

45 Jackson, I.T. & Campbell, J.C. (1970). 'An unusual cause of carpal tunnel syndrome', *J Bone Joint Surg*, **52-B**, 330.

46 Johnson, R.J. & Bonfiglio, M. (1969). 'Lipofibromatous hamartoma of the median nerve', *J Bone Joint Surg*, **51-A**, 984.

47 Jones, H.L. (1895). 'Notes on paralyses of the upper extremity', *St. Bart's Hosp J*, 132.

48 Kaplan, E.B. *Functional and Surgical Anatomy of the Hand* (2nd edition), J.B. Lippincott & Company, Philadelphia, 1972.
49 Kenzora, J.E. (1978). 'Dialysis carpal tunnel syndrome', *Orthopaedics*, **1(3)**, 195.
50 Kilgore, E.S. & Graham, W.P. *The Hand. Surgical and Non-Surgical Treatment*, Lea and Febiger, Philadelphia, 1977.
51 Klofkorn, R.W. & Steigerwald, J.C. (1976). 'Carpal tunnel syndrome as the initial manifestation of tuberculosis', *Am J Med*, **60**, 4.
52 Kojimia, T., Ide, Y., Marumo, E., Ishikawa, E. & Yamashita, H. (1976). 'Haemangioma of the median nerve causing carpal tunnel syndrome', *Hand*, **8**, 62.
53 Kopell, H.P. & Thompson, W.A.L. (1958). 'Pronator syndrome', *N Engl J Med*, **259**, 713.
54 Kopell, H.P. & Thompson, W.A.L. *Peripheral Entrapment Neuropathies*, Williams and Wilkins Company, Baltimore, 1963.
55 Kremer, M., Gilliatt, R.W., Golding, J.S.R. & Wilson, T.G. (1953). 'Acroparaesthesiae in the carpal tunnel syndrome', *Lancet*, **2**, 590.
56 Lamb, D.W. & Kuczynski, K. *The Principles of Hand Surgery*, Blackwell, Oxford, 1981.
57 Lambird, P.A. & Hartmann, W.H. (1969). 'Hereditary amyloidosis, the flexor retinaculum and the carpal tunnel syndrome', *Am J Clin Path*, **52**, 714.
58 Langloh, N.D. & Linscheid, P.L. (1972). 'Recurrent and unrelieved carpal tunnel syndrome', *Clin Orthop*, **83**, 41.
59 Lanz, V. & Volter, J. (1975). 'Das akute carpal tunnel syndrome', *Chirurgie*, **46**, 32.
60 Lanz, U. (1977). 'Anatomical variations of the median nerve in the carpal tunnel', *J Hand Surg*, **2**, 44.
61 Lazaro, L. (1972). 'Carpal tunnel syndrome from insect sting' (A case report), *J Bone Joint Surg*, **54-A**, 1095.
62 Lavey, E.B. & Pearl, R.M. (1981). 'Persistent median artery as a cause of carpal tunnel syndrome', *Ann Plast Surg*, **7**, 236.
63 Learmonth, J.R. (1933). 'The principle of decompression in the treatment of certain diseases of peripheral nerves', *Surg Clin North Am*, **13**, 905.
64 Lettin, A.W.F. (1965). 'Carpal tunnel syndrome in childhood', *J Bone Joint Surg*, **47-B**, 556.
65 Lichtman, D.M., Florio, R.L. & Mack, G.R. (1979). 'Carpal tunnel release under local anesthesia: Evaluation of the outpatient procedure', *J Hand Surg*, **4**, 545.
66 Linscheid, R.L., Peterson, L.F.A. & Juergens, J.L. (1967). 'Carpal tunnel syndrome associated with vasospasm', *J Bone Joint Surg*, **49-A**, 1141.
67 Lipscomb, P.R. (1959). 'Tenosynovitis of the hand and wrist: Carpal tunnel syndrome, de Quervain's disease, trigger digit', *Clin Orthop*, **13**, 164.
68 Lishman, W.A. & Russell, W.R. (1961). 'The brachial neuropathies', *Lancet*, **2**, 941.
69 Marie, P. & Foix, C. (1913). 'Atrophie isolee de l'eminence thenar d'origine nevritique, role du ligament annulaire anterieur du carpe dans la pathogenie de la lesion', *Revue Neurol*, **21**, 647.
70 McCormack, R.M. (1960). 'Carpal tunnel syndrome', *SCNA*, **40**, 517.
71 McLain, E.J. & Wissinger, H.A. (1976). 'The acute carpal tunnel syndrome: nine case reports', *J Trauma*, **16**, 75.
72 Macdonald, R.I. *et al.* (1978). 'Complications of surgical release for carpal tunnel syndrome', *J Hand Surg*, **3**, 70.
73 McLellan, D.L. & Swash, M. (1976). 'Longitudinal sliding of the median nerve during movements of the upper limb', *J Neurol Neurosurg Psychiatry*, **39**, 566.
74 Mangani, U. (1961). 'Some remarks on the etiology of the carpal tunnel compression of the median nerve', *Bull Hosp Joint Dis*, **22**, 56.
75 Mannerfelt, L. & Lund, O.N. (1969). 'Attrition ruptures of flexor tendons in rheumatoid arthritis caused by bony spurs in the carpal tunnel', *J Bone Joint Surg*, **51-B**, 270.
76 Moersch, F.P. (1938). 'Median thenar neuritis. Proceedings Staff Meeting', *Mayo Clin Proc*, **13**, 220.
77 Murley, A.H.G. (1964). 'Orthopaedic surgery in the treatment of leprosy', *J Bone Joint Surg*, **46-B**, 503.
78 Murray, L.C.T. & Wright, V. (1976). 'Carpal tunnel syndrome, humeral epicondylitis and the cervical spine: a study of clinical and dimensional relationship', *Brit Med J*, **1**, 1439.
79 Nicholas, G.G., Noone, B. & Graham, W.P. (1971). 'Carpal tunnel syndrome in pregnancy', *Hand*, **3**, 80.
80 Paget, J. *Lectures on Surgical Pathology* (p. 43), Longman, Brown, Green, Longman, London, 1853.
81 Pecket, P., Gloobe, H. & Nathan, H. (1973). 'Variations in the arteries of the median nerve. With special considerations on the ischemic factor in the carpal tunnel syndrome', *Clin Orthop*, **97**, 144.
82 Phalen, G.S. (1966). 'The carpal tunnel syndrome. Seventeen years experience in diagnosis and treatment of six hundred fifty-four hands', *J Bone Joint Surg*, **48-A**, 211.
83 Phalen, G.S. (1972). 'The carpal tunnel syndrome. Clinical evaluation of 598 hands', *Clin Orthop*, **83**, 29.
84 Phalen, G.S. (1981). 'The birth of a syndrome, or carpal tunnel revisited', *J Hand Surg*, **6**, 109.
85 Phalen, G.S., Gardner, W.J. & La Londe, A.A. (1950). 'Neuropathy of the median nerve due to compression beneath the transverse carpal ligament', *J Bone Joint Surg*, **32-A**, 109.
86 Reid, S.F. (1956). 'Tenovaginitis stenosans at the carpal tunnel', *Aust NZ J Surg*, **25**, 204.
87 Roaf, R. (1947). 'Compression of median nerve in carpal tunnel', *Lancet*, **1**, 387.
88 Robbins, H. (1963). 'Anatomical study of the median nerve in the carpal tunnel and etiologies of the carpal tunnel syndrome', *J Bone Joint Surg*, **45-A**, 953.
89 Sabour, M.S. & Fadel, H.E. (1970). 'The carpal tunnel syndrome – a new complication ascribed to the "pill"', *Am J Obstet Gynecol*, **107**, 1265.
90 Schiller, F. & Kolb, F.O. (1954). 'Carpal tunnel syndrome in acromegaly', *Neurology*, **4**, 271.
91 Sedal, L., McLeod, J.G. & Walsh, J.C. (1973). 'Ulnar nerve lesions associated with the carpal tunnel syndrome', *J Neurol Neurosurg Psychiatry*, **36**, 118.
92 Seddon, H.J. (1952). 'Carpal ganglion as a cause of paralysis of the deep branch of the ulnar nerve', *J Bone Joint Surg*, **34-B**, 386.
93 Semple, J.C. & Cargill, A.O. (1969). 'Carpal tunnel syndrome. Results of surgical decompression', *Lancet*, **1**, 918.
94 Simpson, J.A. (1956). 'Electrical signs in the diagnosis of carpal tunnel and related syndromes', *J Neurol Neurosurg Psychiatry*, **19**, 275.

95 Smith, E.M., Sonstegard, D.A. & Anderson, W.H. Jun. (1977). 'Carpal tunnel syndrome: contribution of flexor tendons', *Arch Phys Med Rehabil*, **58**, 379.
96 Struthers, J. (1849). 'On a peculiarity of the humerus and humeral artery', *Monthly Journal of Medical Science*, **9**, 264.
97 Sunderland, S. (1965). 'The connective tissues of peripheral nerves', *Brain*, **88**, 841.
98 Sunderland, S. *Nerves and Nerve Injuries*, Livingstone, Edinburgh, 1968.
99 Sunderland, S. (1976). 'The nerve lesion in the carpal tunnel syndrome', *J Neurol Neurosurg Psychiatry*, **39**, 615.
100 Spinner, M. *Injuries to the Major Branches of Peripheral Nerves of Forearm*, Saunders, London, 1978.
101 Taleisnik, J. (1973). 'The palmar cutaneous branch of the median nerve and the approach to the carpal tunnel', *J Bone Joint Surg*, **55-A**, 1212.
102 Tanzer, R.C. (1959). 'The carpal tunnel syndrome, a clinical and anatomical study', *J Bone Joint Surg*, **41-A**, 626.
103 Tanzer, R.C. (1959). 'The carpal tunnel syndrome', *Clin Orthop*, **15**, 171.
104 Taylor, A.R. (1974). 'Ulnar compression at the wrist in rheumatoid arthritis', *J Bone Joint Surg*, **56-B**, 142.
105 Upton, A.R. & McComas, A.J. (1973). 'The double crush in nerve entrapment syndromes', *Lancet*, **2**, 359.
106 Vainio, K. (1957). 'Carpal tunnel syndrome caused by tenosynovitis', *Acta Rheum Scand*, **4**, 22.
107 Ward, L.E., Bickel, W.H. & Corbin, K.B. (1958). 'Median neuritis (carpal tunnel syndrome) caused by gouty tophi', *J Am Med Assoc*, **167**, 844.
108 Warren, D.J. & Otieno, L.S. (1975). 'Carpal tunnel syndrome in patients on intermittent haemodialysis', *Postgrad Med J*, **51**, 540.
109 Wartenberg, R. (1939). 'Partial thenar atrophy. A clinical entity', *Arch Neurol Psychiatry*, **42**, 373.
110 Wood, C. (1961). 'Paraesthesia of the hand in pregnancy', *Brit Med J*, **2**, 681.
111 Wynn-Parry, C.B. *Strength duration curves. In Lichts. Electrodiagnosis and electromyography*, Licht, Newhaven, Conn., 1962.

Miscellaneous Tables

Table 13. Carpal tunnel syndrome

Sex: F/M, 5/1.

Age: 30–60 years

Occupation: Repetitive use of fingers and wrist; e.g. housewife, process worker, etc.

Mostly dominant hand. Bilateral in 50 per cent

Associated hand conditions, e.g. flexor tenosynovitis, flexor tenovaginitis, rheumatoid disease

Associated general conditions, e.g. diabetes mellitus, pregnancy, menopause, myxoedema, etc.

Table 14. Carpal tunnel syndrome – four key questions to ask

1 Is this carpal tunnel syndrome?

2 What is the likely cause?

3 Are there associated conditions?

4 Is conservative or is operative treatment indicated?

Table 15. Pathogenesis of carpal tunnel syndrome (CTS)

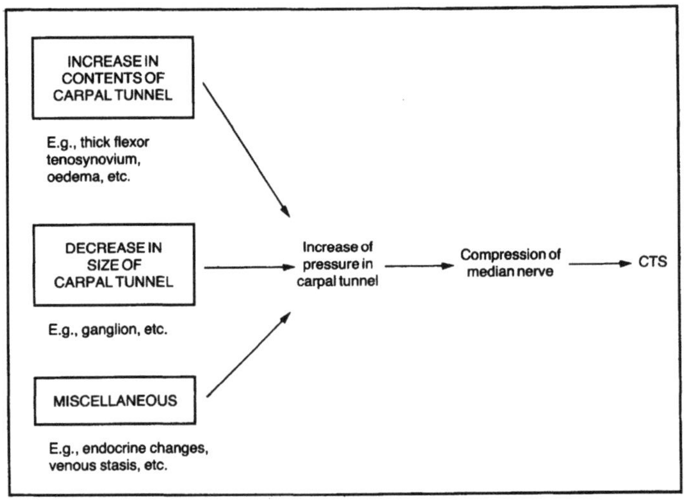

Table 16. Diagnosis of carpal tunnel syndrome

Symptoms	Signs†	Investigations
Pain, paraesthesiae (worse at night*, relieved by hand exercise) Weakness/clumsiness (worse in the morning, usually passes off during the day unless unusual manual activity is undertaken with the wrist flexed)	Impaired sensation Tinel's sign Phalen's test Thenar tenderness or weakness	Xray (carpal tunnel view) EMG delay of sensory and/or motor conduction

*'Waking numbness' is diagnostic of CTS.
†In about one-third to one-fourth there are no abnormal signs.
‡Most cases of CTS can be diagnosed by history and examination.
EMG is said to be accurate in 80 to 90 per cent, but the test is not necessary in most cases.

Table 17. Carpal tunnel decompression – surgical technique

1 Tourniquet and hand surgery facilities
2 Incise parallel to and on ulnar side of thenar crease from mid-palm to the wrist crease
3 Expose the superficial palmar arch distally and then deepen the dissection to expose the flexor retinaculum
4 Incise the flexor retinaculum on the ulnar side of the midline. Protect the median nerve
5 Expose the median nerve and identify its five terminal sensory and its recurrent thenar motor branch. Beware of anomalies
6 Divide the proximal and distal attachments of the flexor retinaculum, e.g. deep fascia of forearm
7 Note the condition of the median nerve – see indications for external and internal neurolysis, etc.
8 Examine the carpal tunnel for signs of a space-occupying lesion
9 Close the skin wound with fine interrupted sutures
10 Apply a standard non-adherent compressive hand dressing
11 Splint the wrist with a plaster slab

Table 18. Carpal tunnel decompression. Causes of failure[56, 72]

Causes of failure	Prevention
1 Incorrect or delay in diagnosis	Careful clinical assessment
2 Iatrogenic injury (e.g. to median nerve or its branches) 3 Inadequate decompression	Interthenar exposure 'under vision'
4 Postoperative • pain • swelling • stiffness	Splint the wrist Exercise the fingers
5 Postoperative • fibrosis in carpal tunnel	Precise surgical technique (haemostasis) splint the wrist for 2 weeks
6 Recurrent tenosynovitis	Tenosynovectomy for significant bulk or invasive tenosynovitis

Index

Figures in medium type indicate page numbers; those in **bold** indicate figure numbers.

U

V

W

X

Bei Fragen zur Produktsicherheit wenden Sie sich bitte an:
If you have any questions regarding product safety,
please contact:

Walter de Gruyter GmbH
Genthiner Straße 13
10785 Berlin
productsafety@degruyterbrill.com